Lymphedema Warriors
Health & Wellness

Complete Decongestive Therapy, Exercises & Nutrition.

Dr. Ivy Sardoncillo-Enting

Physical Therapist and Certified Lymphedema Therapist

DISCLAIMER

The information in this book is for educational purposes on lymphedema. Its pathophysiology, risks factors, incidence, and possible treatment coupled with scientific evidence through research, experiences by the author as a clinician and stories, and hands-on experiences by the lymphedema patients.

The stories highlighted in this book are not specific to a client. No names, no locations are written. All information is taken from past experiences of the writer on this topic while treating the medical issue.

All pictures, images, and illustrations in the book have proper consent from the creators.

The book is for information only and does not warrant a treatment book, nor is it intended as a substitute for medical advice, even though the writer is a Doctor of Physical Therapy and a Certified Lymphedema Therapist. It is highly recommended that the reader has a regular and proper consult by a health care provider, particularly on signs and symptoms related to the topic of this book.

Lastly, do not follow the treatment recommended in this book without proper diagnosis and assessment by your medical providers. All of the pertinent information in this book is for general knowledge and understanding only.

DEDICATION

I dedicate this book to the people who made it possible. I would not have been able to do this without their help and support. To all lymphedema patients whom I get to see and talk and educate on how to deal and fight this condition, and how to live a normal life and to keep going no matter what, this book is for you, to hopefully inspire you to keep the fight and be a warrior in your everyday existence, and to be an inspiration to your family, to your community and to the whole world.

To all cancer patients with lymphedema complications, I am hoping this book can help you in little ways of understanding yourself in this situation and be able to continue the fight of both the cancer and the lymphedema and to always keep in mind and heart that you are bigger and stronger than these two horrendous conditions.

ABOUT THE AUTHOR

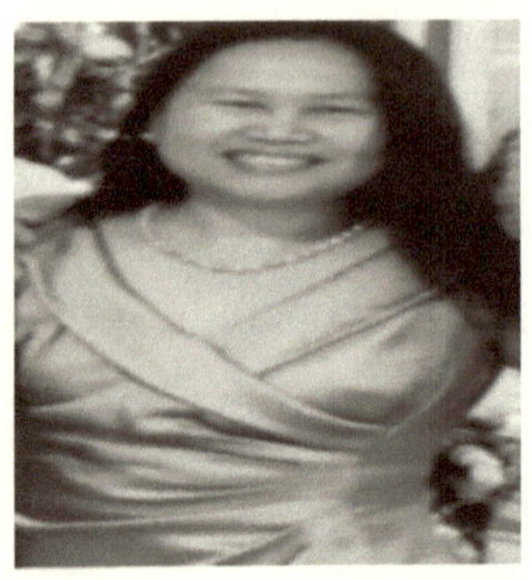

Dr. Ivy Sardoncillo Enting is a Doctor of Physical Therapy. She is also a certified lymphedema therapist and a certified wound debridement therapist, a certified LSVT BIG physical therapist for people with Parkinson's disease. She is also a vestibular therapist. Dr. Ivy sees geriatric and middle-aged clients in the home health setting as well as through phone and video consultations as needed with various physical therapy and lymphedema needs.

Recently, Ivy works primarily as a home health physical therapist in the Tampa Bay area Florida. She is the co-owner of Rivyve Therapy Services LLC. The owner of Smart & Caring PhysioDoc online services.

Ivy loves to write anything about health & wellness and physical therapy. She also loves family personal finance topics. You can read her blogs at her website "Smart & Caring PhysioDoc, Pay It Forward." She offers telehealth physical therapy consultations for health and wellness and physical therapy evaluation and treatment for cases including but not limited to lymphedema cases, Parkinson's disease, and pain-related movement issues for her remote clients via computer-based or video conferencing method.

She is from the Queen City of the South, in the beautiful Island of the Philippines. A country located in the pacific with 7,700 plus lovely islands during low tide, and recently with mother nature, keep on shaking and shifting the earth, adding more islets for the natives to enjoy.

Ivy was born in a progressing country that majority of the people have to work in order to eat and live to enjoy the basics of life. Her parents worked so hard to put food in the table. Her father was an electrician who provides houses and buildings the electricity, but ironically, she quoted, "we don't have electricity at home. However, we have kerosene lamps, and of course, candles to give us light during the nighttime."

Her childhood was spent happily in the Philippines. It has been her dream to one day be able to live comfortably in a fully functioning home with lights and electricity and no leaky roof. She is not only a dreamer but a firm believer that if there is a will, there is always a way. And that poverty is never going to be a hindrance of for anyone's success. With prayers and faith and hard work, everything is possible.

She finished her bachelor's degree in Physical Therapy at Southwestern University, a prestigious university in Cebu City, Philippines. Ivy has been a physical therapist since 1997 and worked in different settings, from being a clinical instructor to working in the hospital and outpatient and home health setting in her native country, Philippines.

She migrated to the United States of America in October of 2008 and has worked in Sarasota, Florida, in the skilled nursing home facilities. Ivy got certified for lymphedema therapy from the Academy of Lymphatic Studies in 2011. Became a vestibular therapist in 2016, and LSVT BIG certified on 2017. Dr. Ivy fulfilled her longtime dream of becoming a Doctor of Physical Therapy by furthering her study at Utica College, New York, and graduated in May 2017.

Ivy loves her country of birth as much as she loves her second home, the beautiful land of milk and honey, the great United States of America.

"Life in the United States of America, is so beautiful and full of great opportunities to anyone who wants to move up in life."I.E

TABLE OF CONTENTS

10

FOREWORD

<u>**Dr. Lohindren Adorable**</u>

*Physiatrist, Dean of the College of Rehabilitation
Sciences, Southwestern University, Philippines*

I have known Ivy Sardoncillo-Enting for two decades now. The first decade was the most significant as she and I worked together in the same university rehabilitation clinic where I am being the physiatrist, evaluated and medically managed patients and referred them to her subsequently for physical therapy. His extraordinary technical and people skills made me decide as a dean also of the university's college of rehabilitative sciences to assign her physical therapy interns, so they can learn her style and multiply the likes of her in the next generation of the physical therapist. Her departure from our country to work and study in the US marked the start of the second decade. In this period, she continues to connect with us in all media to support and share ideas on how to improve further the physical therapy profession in the country, including the putting up of the first DPT program in the region and the development of specialties like wound and lymphedema therapy.

With the author's very formidable roots and broad-based background in the practice of the profession, there is an assurance that this book will benefit PT students and clinicians, especially those practicing this specialty, the medical and allied healthcare practitioners, the patients and anyone in the community.

In our university, and in our country, this will surely be a prime reference book. So, there should be no reason that others would have second thoughts in getting a copy of this book.

<u>Denise M. McVay, PT, DPT</u>

Board Certified Clinical Specialist in Geriatric Physical Therapy (GCS)

Director, Post-professional tDPT Program

Utica College, Utica, NY

As the Director and faculty member of a Post-professional (transitional) Doctor of Physical Therapy program, I have known the author for many years as one of our former successful doctoral program graduates. The author's impetus in writing this work is to share with the reader the stories and experiences-the wins and hopes-of all patients

13

and clients she has worked with on her journey as a physical therapist and specifically, a physical therapist working with patients/clients who have lymphedema, as well as those who are cancer survivors. The author makes it clear that she was compelled to complete this work as she derives inspiration from and has the highest respect of all of her patients.

For several years, the author has demonstrated an unending passion for those persevering through the effects of lymphedema-its complications, treatments, etc. The author has written the book primarily as an informational journey, discussing aspects of lymphedema such as cause, risks, prognosis and treatment, and includes stories of lymphedema warriors and their families and caregivers. She has also made sure to include evidence-based support for the information provided, to paint a clearer picture of the medical condition that has come to be known as one of the leading causes of financial, physical, social and emotional burden for many who are affected.

This book is particularly important as a means to offer hope to those seeking assistance with the effects of lymphedema. This work, a 'go-to' book of sorts, is not intended as a treatment book, but rather a testimony to understand lymphedema, including treatment, prevention, exercises, self -management and other aspects about this medical condition, supported by evidence-based clinical research of all pertinent therapies.

This book is written to honor all of the lymphedema patients and cancer survivors that the author has had the privilege to work with over these many years, and I invite you to enjoy this work as you, your family members and any others experiencing the effects of lymphedema, move forward to reach your personal goals.

<u>Karen Mooney-Crouch, RN, NY</u>

"I alone cannot change the world, but I can cast a stone across the waters to create many ripples", Mother Teresa

To the readers of this book:
Compassion and touching other people's life is what Ivy Enting does through her advanced knowledge of physical therapy. I met Ivy while working as a Home Health Coordinator. Coordinating care for patients was an absolute

15

pleasure when I had the best physical therapist to work alongside in my 20 plus year healthcare career, knowing my patients had Ivy as their physical therapist. I have worked in many healthcare settings in my career but working with Ivy in the home health care setting set the bar much higher. Ivy's dedication to the whole patient and her enthusiasm to learn, teach and treat her patients surpasses any other I've known. Her eagerness to learn and master the art of physical therapy and the benefits to her patients is amazing. It was such an honor to be a part of the team working with Ivy.

<u>**Cherryl Balansag Concha, PT**</u>

Physical Therapist Sunterrace Skilled Nursing Rehabilitation facility Sun City Center Florida, and former director of Rehabilitation at Shore Acres Rehabilitation Center St Petersburg Florida

"Happy is the man that findeth wisdom and the man that getteth understanding. " Proverbs 3:13

A book to be worth reading must do more than amuse and interest. It must be instructive to be of real value to the reader. The study of lymphedema is a many-sided subject.

16

With this view, the author has endeavored to make the following work as complete and practical as limited space would allow. Constant practice and persistent application of the rules outlined will be worth the effort expended. Patience, practice, and perseverance, together with a spirit of happiness in one's work, are bound to bring the rich rewards that a world of opportunity offers. I personally have known Dr. Ivy Enting, the author, for at least 20 years. She has been my constant companion and mentor since my Physical Therapy Internship. I have witnessed her exemplary work and excellence in the field of Physical Therapy as she has shown positive outcome and touched others' lives, her being authentic, and always open to receiving as well as giving, it is a good description of many of the most amazing people I've encountered. As a clinician, I expect this book will quickly become an easy 'standard reference' on lymphedema as the clinical information is concise, thorough, and up-to-date.

Mr. Leo Euraoba, MBA, MSCTS

Masters in Computer Science and Teaching, Government Consultant in IT Department of Saskatchewan, Canada

I have known the author for more than four years in her university days and another ten years in her professional work as a Physiotherapist. As one of the university professors at Southwestern University, she has shown unwavering dedication and commitment to her studies. She is always top-notch in her Physical Therapy classes. Ivy Sardoncillo-Enting is a born leader. Graduated valedictorian in High School and a Dean's lister in her university days. She motivates her team members to work with peers as well as working hard on their own. She is a good listener but at home and work. I have seen her rise from poverty to a successful investor. I do not doubt that she is exceptionally qualified to write a book on health and wellness.

As a consultant for the government of the Saskatchewan IT Division in Canada, I know how she uses the latest technology and techniques in the application of her field of study. I gave my 100 percent support in her desire to write a book on "Lymphedema Warriors Health & Wellness." Be prepared to explore the myriad of principles and techniques found in this book.

ACKNOWLEDGEMENTS

I am thankful for the blessings that Our Almighty God has bestowed on me in giving me the knowledge and dedication to write this book to share with everyone that needs the information and to help them live their lives to the fullest.

To my husband, Enrico Jr., who inspires me to keep pushing in reaching my dreams and aspirations. To my children Franque, Gerard, and Rita Mae, who are my number one fans and cheerers, who always believe in me that I can pursue my dreams for myself, for them and for all the people that I love to serve.

To my book Boss mentor, Dr. Jeremy Sutton, PT, thank you for believing that I and all of us in the HSPA academy are authors in our ways. You can follow him on his website www.healthybooks.net.

I would like to acknowledge the friends and colleagues that made this book possible.

To all my clients and all lymphedema warriors, this book is dedicated to you all in the hopes of making your fight a little easy and light.

I am so grateful for the kind and uplifting words written in the Foreword section of this book from my professors, colleagues and mentors, namely:

Dr. Lohindren Adorable, physiatrist and Dean of Southwestern University/Phinma College of Rehabilitation Services and Sports Sciences.

Denise M. McVay, PT, DPT
Board Certified Clinical Specialist in Geriatric Physical Therapy (GCS), Director, Post-professional tDPT Program, Utica College, Utica, NY

Mr. Leo Euraoba, the head consultant for the government of Saskatchewan IT Division in Canada.

Mrs. Cherryl Balansag-Concha, lead Physical Therapist of Sunterrace Rehabilitation Center of Sun City Center, Florida.

Karen Mooney-Crouch, Registered Nurse, NY.

Former Director of Sales and marketing for Nurse on Call
Tampa Florida.

INTRODUCTION

I am super excited to write this book to understand lymphedema simply, coupled with research-and-clinical based pieces of evidence. To hopefully have the readers see a clear picture of the medical condition.

I am very inspired to get this book written and published to share the experiences, the wins, and the hopes of all the clients that I had in my journey as a physical therapist and a lymphedema therapist. The highest respect and inspiration that I gained from all of the lymphedema and cancer survivor clients are enough to give me the overpowering urge to write this book. The title of the book was derived from this inspiration, and to the respect of the warriors referenced here.

To share their stories, paint a clear picture of the medical condition that has become known at present as one of the leading causes of a financial, physical, social and emotional burden to some that are affected.

Besides, creating a simple to-go book on understanding about lymphedema, its treatment, prevention, exercises, self - management, and everything and anything we should know about this medical condition.

The book talks about lymphedema and its pertinent information from its causes, risks, prognosis, and treatment. It tells about the stories of the lymphedema warriors, and their families and caregivers who are the main spotlight of why the author wrote this book.

The book is for information only and does not warrant a treatment manual. Do not follow the treatment recommended here without proper diagnosis and assessment by your medical providers. All of the pertinent information in this book is for general knowledge and understanding only.

For a more detailed evaluation and management, one is highly advised to seek professional consultation from your physician, Doctor of Physical Therapy, primary care doctor, or from a certified lymphedema therapist.

BECOMING A LYMPHEDEMA WARRIOR

Life is a cycle.

On the eastern side of the globe, one wakes up with the sun's beautiful rays rising. While on the opposite western front, one sleeps as the magical sun's radiant light sets and swims down into the ocean's depth. With every ticking of the clock, one is born and breathes in their first air that makes one happy and gay. And sadly, one also dies and gasps their last breath of air as the beauty of their eyes slowly closes as the warrior of death takes them home.

One day we are healthy and full of energy, and the next day, we are devoid of this power and fuel to get going with life.

But men get up after each fall, rises every time they fall. No matter how hard the fall, humans manage to stand up and continue to the hustle and bustle and live life to the fullest.

The human race is unique. It is born to make an impact on society. It is part of the musculoskeletal system of the world that poses different roles. We have our own unique and distinct character that makes the earth the most livable planet on the solar system. Some are stronger in their physical wellness, others on their emotional and mental wellness. No human being is perfect, but we have an ideal world that makes each one plays a part of the team. That is why no man is an island.

Humans are like the warriors we see in the movies. Going down through memory lane the history of our existence, from the stories in the Bible to the first World War to the second to Vietnam and then the Korean wars, our scientists and medical health experts have continuously searched for the perfect weapons on the fight to end diseases. These viruses and bacteria are leading causes of deadly and incurable diseases that constantly wreak havoc in the health and wellness landscape of life.

The healthcare professionals are not the only soldiers on the ground, but all human beings are part of the whole team. We are all considered warriors in the fight for freedom, peace, and health and wellness globally.

Plenty of people of different age categories are becoming more engaged and empowered with lifestyle changes through exercises, diet and proper nutrition, mental and emotional health and wellness programs.

Nowadays, young and old alike are pretty much engaged in sports, potpourri of exercises suitable to one's choice, becoming a member of their favorite gym, and participating in community activities. Some loves to run a marathon, do road or mountain biking, and others engulf themselves in tri-sports. The communing to the health and wellness of the society has gained popularity with the advent of new genres.

Commonly, a lot of tech geniuses are inventing virtual exercises to keep up with the busy lifestyle for some Gen-Xers, millennials and baby boomers both to generate passive financial income and as well as to improve their health and wellness. Hitting two birds with one golden stone, it is!

It is not just a trend in this techy genre but a way of life due to the increasingly sedentary lifestyle brought by this highly machine-operated and robotics' new world, which enhances the rise in the percentage of the obesity epidemic in the global world.

The majority of us are becoming warriors in living the ultimate disease-proof life, in the hopes of such a phenomenon will become a reality in the future of our world.

Have we considered what is on the other side of the spectrum? *What do you think is happening on the tail-end or head side of the coin?*

The people that are on the side of having issues of unhealthiness or poor-health brought by numerous diseases and illnesses, which includes one of the most remarkable increases in body mass index leading to obesity syndrome. Obesity affects the physical, emotional and mental wellness of an individual.

The continued pursuit of the world's search for the perfect exercise, diet, and lifestyle modification is far worse in this group. It is compromised if the person searching for the utmost remedy has some medical comorbidities relatable to

27

obesity or overweight such as lymphedema or they are living or born with lymphedema. The relationship between obesity and lymphedema will be given emphasis in the later chapter of this book.

Each one of us is warriors in the fight of our lives. The lymphedema warriors, the cancer-survivor warriors, and people with lymphedema are warriors living in their unique condition and situation. It is indeed a constant fight in the hopes that one day; they will be on the brighter side of the spectrum and enjoy their lives within normal limits of their health and wellness. And be able to fully appreciate and function despite some inabilities; and be just like anyone that is not in the same war they're in, and who are not wearing the same lymph boots, they are wearing.

"Courage, above all things, is the first quality of a warrior." Karl von Clau

CHAPTER 1

UNDERSTANDING LYMPHEDEMA

What makes this condition unique and needs special attention and better understanding?

What causes my leg, arm, belly, and private parts to swell? What makes my skin thicker and harder? Is this curable? How did I get this? These are a few of the many questions I have heard from my clients that came to see me for this problem.

To better understand the condition is to learn what is the normal function of the body system that is being affected by lymphedema. We have learned earlier in high school or perhaps middle school years, the arterial and venous system as the main component of the circulatory system in addition to the heart. Later on, we learn about the lymphatic system. Let us get to know the two systems here.

The circulatory system is a closed system, where the veins supply blood without oxygen or the blue blood from the systemic circulation, and the arteries supply the blood with oxygen or the red blood from the heart to be distributed throughout the body organs or to the systemic circulation.

Circulatory system

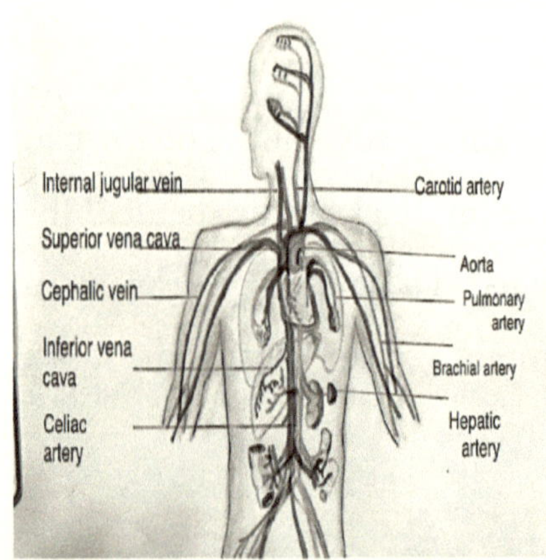

Image is from the sketch drawing of EE (Enrico Enting) with permission.

The illustration below shows the healthy circulation of the veins and arteries to and from the heart. It emphasizes the close circuit circulation.

HEART
LUNGS
ARTERIES/RED BLOOD WITH O2
CAPILLARIES
BODY PARTS/ O2 ABSORBED AS NUTRIENTS
VEINS/BLUE BLOOD WITH NO O2

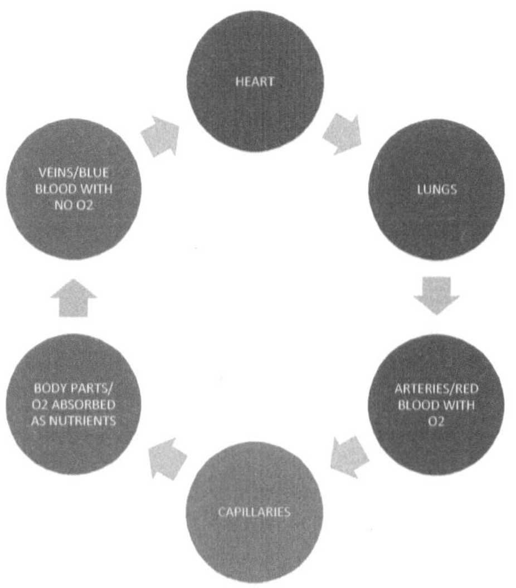

31

Below is a complete blood circulation from the Oxygen poor blood to the oxygen-rich blood.

Oxygen-poor blood returns from the body to the heart through the superior vena cava and inferior vena cava

Oxygen-poor blood enters the right atrium, (right upper chamber of the heart).

Blood flows through the tricuspid valve into the right ventricle(right lower chamber of the heart).

RV pumps oxygen-poor blood through the pulmonary valve into the main pulmonary artery.

Then the blood flows through the right and left pulmonary arteries into the LUNGS.

During breathing inside the lungs. Oxygen sent to the blood and Carbon dioxide is taken out of the blood. OXYGEN- RICH blood

Oxygen-rich blood flows from the lungs back into the left atrium (left upper chamber of the heart) through four pulmonary vein

Oxygen-rich blood then flows through the mitral valve into the left ventricle (the left lower chamber).

Left ventricle pumps the oxygen-rich blood , through the aortic valve into the aorta the main artery that takes oxygen-rich blood out to the rest of the body.

The lymphatic system on the other hand is developed as an offshoot of the venous system that consists of lymph vessels, lymph nodes, and lymph ducts that transport lymph fluid throughout the body and is an open system.

Lymphatic system

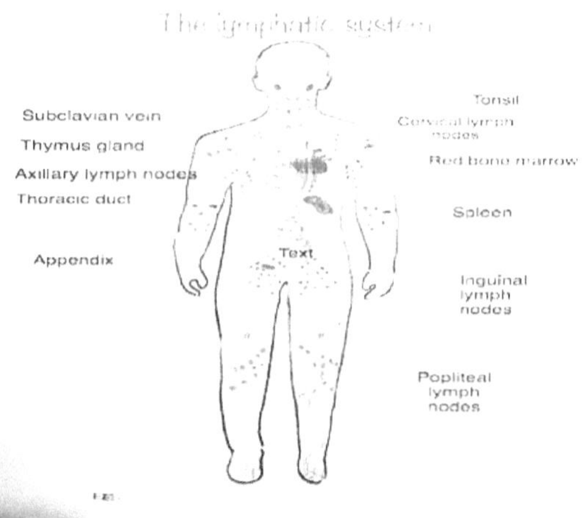

Image is *from* *the sketch drawing of EE (Enrico Enting) with permission.*

Blood from the arteries/capillaries/veins in a closed circuit. Lymph flows in an open circuit from the tissues to the lymphatic vessels.

33

Table comparison between two the systems.

Circulatory system	Lymphatic system
Blood flows from arteries, to the capillaries and to the veins and back to the heart. It is a close circuit. Supplies nutrients through oxygenated blood to the cells of the body	Lymph flows in an open circuit from the lymphatic vessels, lymphatic trunk, collecting ducts, veins bloodstreams. It is an open circuit. Flows in one direction only towards the heart. Functions for absorption, immune system and fluid balance.

The illustration below is the flow of lymph fluid within the lymphatic system.

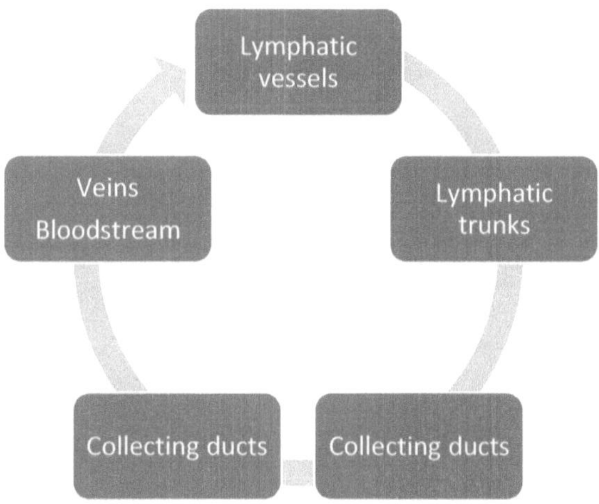

What are the essential functions of the lymphatic system? The lymphatic system helps in removing excess fluids from body tissues (fluid homeostasis), it absorbs fatty acids and transport fats in the digestive system, and it produces immune cells to fight infections in the body.

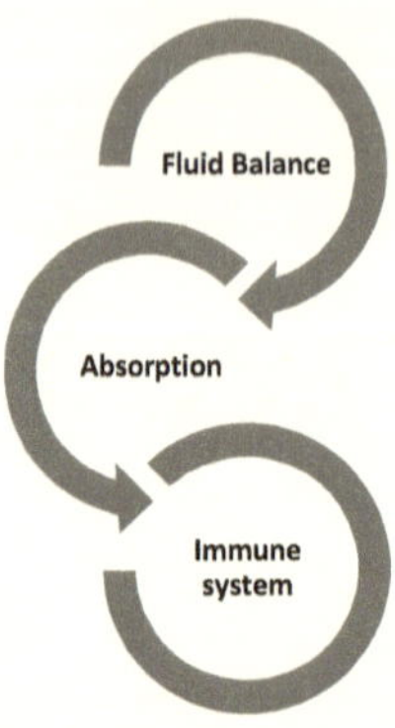

The above image illustrates the three important functions of the lymphatic system:

Fluid balance (removes excess proteins and fluid from the tissues)

Absorption (fatty acids in the gut)

Immune system (defense mechanism against unwanted organisms).

So, what is lymphedema then?

> "A medical condition which is an abnormal swelling of the extremity(limb) due to the failure of the lymphatic system to eliminate or get rid of lymph fluid into the circulation."

It is a condition that affects the lymphatic system due to an injury or malfunction of the system. Lymphedema is a combination of the words lymph + edema (lymph a clear protein-rich fluid of the lymphatic system and edema or swelling). It is due to an abnormal build-up of protein-rich fluid in the outside of the tissue cells of the body.

According to the National Lymphedema Network, the primary acquired or hereditary, is where the lymphatic vessels are missing or impaired. The primary or congenital LE is from "aplasia or hypoplasia," absence or diminished lymphatic system. It is primary or congenital, meaning you have it, or it's developed or born with you. Some say it's genetic.

The second group is the secondary lymphedema such as postmastectomy lymphedema, edema or swelling after replacement surgery, abdominal surgery, or any surgeries that cause injury to the lymphatic system. The secondary type is also due to a damage to the lymph vessels or removal of lymph nodes that are not uncommon among cancer surgical procedures.

The most common example of this type is the postmastectomy lymphedema after removal of breasts and axillary lymph nodes from cancer of the breasts and for the

lower extremity or leg edema from surgical removal of
inguinal lymph nodes of the groin and popliteal lymph
nodes from the back of the knee from different causes. The
upper arms, forearm, hand and legs, abdomen, trunk, head
and neck, genitals, and inner organs of the body can be
affected with lymphedema.

Through my experience in treating lymphedema patients,
and in talking to them of how they feel about their condition,
I have gathered that the majority of them are embarrassed
about the appearance of their skin. The majority are scared or
afraid to go out in public. Lymphedema is becoming as one
of the leading causes of social embarrassment due to skin
integrity issues and swollen limbs.

Not everyone living with this condition is equipped with
the knowledge in what to do and how to get rid of the issues
brought by this. Also, not all medical professionals are aware
of the condition and always connote this to the obesity issue.

I still remember during the earlier days(eight years ago)
as a practicing physical therapy specialist in lymphedema
therapy, we have to do marketing to some doctors that do not

have a thorough knowledge of the disease and its appropriate treatment or remedies. Not all physicians are on board on the issues. Their first line of defense when this group of patients sees them is by prescribing the famous" water pill."

So, if not all medical professional is aware and knowledgeable of the condition, then this makes it more difficult for the person having the disease to understand his or her health issue. Therefore, proper teaching and education about lymphedema is not only a necessity in the family level but also in the community as well.

"Hear it from the lymphedema warriors".

Some say, my arms, legs, or stomach is big and fat, or they are swollen because I overeat salty foods. "I overeat." I love hamburgers, pasta and potato fries. But is this the reason why I have a swollen leg or arm, belly, or even my genitals are puffy.

One young-elderly woman came to see me in the clinic for an assessment of her right leg swelling. She said, "My leg started swelling after we went hiking in the woods and bug

39

bites, feasted on my legs, then after a few days, my right leg started to get sore and bigger."

Other stories, "My leg started swelling after I sustained a skin tear from a fall at home that did not heal quickly. Another client foretold her story stating, "My doctor said I don't have lymphedema, my legs are just full of fat because I am morbidly obese."

The most common reason people see me for lymphedema therapy is due to the postmastectomy procedure for breast cancer. They comprise fifty percent of the clients that I treat. Another huge group of clients I take care of, are obesity-related lymphedema complicated by comorbidities such as diabetes mellitus, high blood pressure, obesity, sedentary lifestyle, kidney problems, heart failure, anemia, and other fluid retention issues.

A very popular question is "How will I know if I have true lymphedema or a false one"? And when to see a lymphedema therapist.

Let me present three scenarios that are not uncommon in clinical practice.

Scenario 1: *A charming lady who came to see me for the assessment and management of her right leg edema who presented with both lower legs swelling, right is more pronounced than the left. She is a young, elderly 68-year-old lady who is 68 inches in height and weighs 175 pounds. Pertinent medical histories include hypertension, diabetes mellitus, right knee total arthroplasty two years ago, low back pain, and hysterectomy, and appendectomy. Her chief complaint is swelling of her right leg that doesn't go away with elevation and with her taking water pill prescribed by her family doctor. She further narrated her right leg is more swollen at the end of the day and hinders her playing golf as it gets heavy with prolonged walking and standing. She denies pain on her legs but has issues with lower back intermittent aching pain.*

Scenario 2. *A morbidly obese 70-year-old gentleman presented with weeping edema of both lower extremity, and edema of his abdomen. He complains of shortness of breath (SOB) upon exertion, pain on both knees in prolonged* *standing, and difficulty in lower body dressing and shower activities. Pertinent medical histories include hypertension, prostatic hypertrophy, stage 2 kidney disease, Congestive heart failure, and COPD. He reported that his leg edema slightly subsides in size and volume early morning and when he elevates his leg in the recliner chair.*

Scenario 3. *A delightful 65-year-old lady who is a 5- year postmastectomy client came to see me for an assessment of her armpit edema, both arms and hands swelling and thickened and hardened skin texture. She had histories of radiation therapy after her bilateral mastectomy, had eight lymph nodes removal on her left armpit and 12 in her left armpit. No chemotherapy. She is on remission for five years now. One morning, she woke up and felt tightness and a big lump on her left armpit, and she moved her arms up and down and did all kinds of exercises, and the lump decreased in size. But on the third day, the swelling increased in size, which prompted her to see her primary care physician (PCP). Her PCP referred her to a lymphedema therapist for evaluation and treatment. She has no clue about lymphedema. She was not given any education about lymphedema and its treatment earlier until lately; she went* *to see her PCP for her left armpit swelling. The has postmastectomy lymphedema, which is a very common complication of breast cancer after the removal of the breast and the axillary lymph nodes. She was very thankful for the education on her new issue that was given by her therapist, and it gave her hope that the swelling can be managed with proper training and treatment.*

Now of the three scenarios presented, which do you think has a true lymphedema?

Yes, you are right, scenario #3 has a true lymphedema. She had mastectomy and removal of her axillary lymph nodes, thus there is an injury to her lymphatic system. The scenarios no. 2 and no. 3, the swelling or edema is related to their comorbidities such as CHF, chronic kidney disease, and obesity, and swelling due to replacement surgery.

CHAPTER 2

STAGES AND TYPES OF LYMPHEDEMA

Stages		
0 Latent Pre-stage	↓ lymph transport or circulation	No visible edema
1 Reversible	+ protein rich fluid ↑ edema with heat, humidity and activity	+ pitting edema ↓ edema with elevation, normal size in the AM
2 Irreversible	+ protein rich fluid + nonpitting edema	+ connective scar tissue + clinical fibrosis skin changes
3 Lymphostatic elephantiasis	Severe nonpitting fibrotic edema + protein rich fluid	Hardening of skin tissues, keratosis, hyperpigmentation, ↑ skin folds

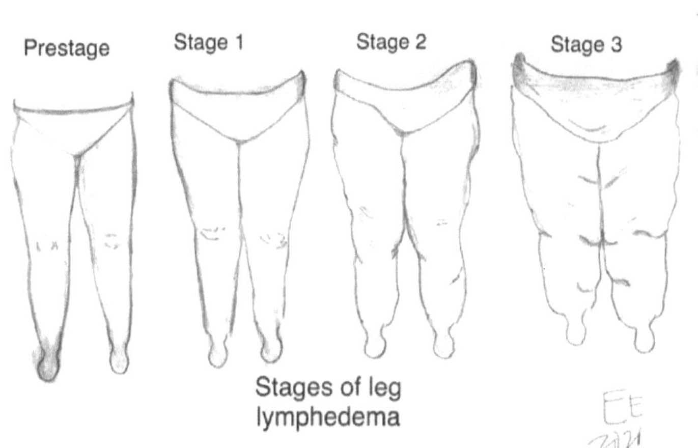

Image is from the sketch drawing of EE (Enrico Enting) with permission.

Lymphedema has two types, they can be either primary or secondary. This means it can occur on its own (primary lymphedema), or it can be caused by another disease or condition (secondary lymphedema). Secondary lymphedema is far more common than primary lymphedema.

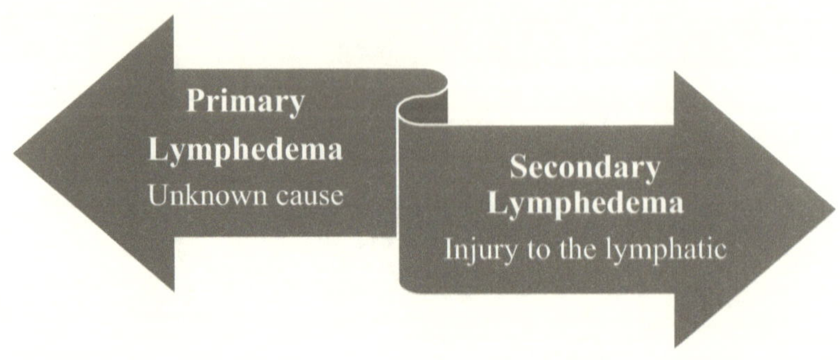

Image is from the sketch drawing of EE (Enrico Enting) with permission.

Above is an illustration and sample images for the Classification of lymphedema.

CHAPTER 3

TREATING LYMPHEDEMA

Becoming a certified lymphedema therapist and allied medical professional, one has to undergo a comprehensive training seminar and hands-on training on anatomy, pathology, physiology, and the treatment of lymphedema. And one has to pass the certification examination of both written and laboratory (hands-on techniques) to get the title of a certified lymphedema therapist and able to treat clients with this medical condition.

When I had my training to become a certified lymphedema therapist in 2011, I still clearly remembered my instructor's quick response to the question, if lymphedema is curable, it was a resounding NO! However, it might not be curable, but it is preventable, that is why we are all here to learn about this condition and make a difference. That gave us all a sigh of relief and built up everyone's curiosity about what we will be dealing with for the 11 days comprehensive training seminar.

The treatment of lymphedema is popularly known as Complete Decongestive Therapy (CDT). The term decongestive is used to decongest or unclog the area of swelling. The main idea of the treatment is to reroute the lymph fluid or edema to the latency or dormant stage by using the remaining intact lymph vessels and using other pathways that are still open.

COMPLETE DECONGESTIVE THERAPY is the gold standard of treatment for LE. It is a noninvasive treatment that comprises manual lymph drainage, compression bandaging, decongestive exercises, and compression stockings or garments that can either be custom-made or regular. In Europe, CDT started in 1970, and in the USA, this became well known in the 1980s.

A complete assessment of the body system is performed to rule out a definitive diagnosis of lymphedema and its causative factor unique for each client. When a comprehensive assessment is finished, then the therapy will

48

commence for the implementation of complete decongestive therapy.

A good example that I frequently use to explain lymphedema therapy to my clients is citing a traffic accident on a highway. If I-75 has a car accident that involves one or more vehicles, the initial effect of such an accident will be congestion in the area before the site. Just like having lymphedema, there will be swelling on the left or right arm from the shoulders down to the fingers, because of an injury or removal of axillary lymph nodes that affect the flow of fluid to the normal circulatory pathway. So, with the car accident in I-75, what the troopers or the EMS does is to guide the other vehicles to an area where there is still a way for the cars to continue and be away from the accident for the traffic to continue to flow. They will reroute the other vehicle to decongest the area.

In lymphedema therapy, the same idea happens. A specially trained, certified lymphedema therapist is the only one that can do the CDT. The majority of the lymphedema therapist undergoes a comprehensive training seminar and has to pass a certification examination to become eligible to treat and assess lymphedema cases.

There are two phases of CDT:

Phases	Treatment
Phase I	The compression treatment to decrease swelling and decongest the area with lymphedema. 1. Skin care 2. Manual lymphatic drainage therapy 3. Decongestive exercises 4. Compression therapy.
Phase II	The self-management/maintenance phase. The goals here is preservation of the results from phase I.

SKIN CARE FOR LYMPHEDEMA

Tips for lymphedema skincare:

1. Avoid injury or trauma to the skin to prevent infection.

2. Keep the affected area clean and dry. Make sure to dry feet and the web of the toes thoroughly. Apply moisturizer daily to prevent chapping and chafing of skin.

3. Do not use lotions with strong smells or odors as they are very acidic.

4. Nail care should be taken cared of properly.

5. Do not have manicurist cut your nails, have the podiatrist do the job. Have podiatrist cut your toe nails to prevent infections.

6. Use insect repellant and sunscreen for exposed skin.

7. When using razors be extra careful to avoid skin irritation.

8. Wear gloves during activities such as gardening, working with tools, washing dishes that can cause skin injury.

9. Contact your primary physician immediately if you have rashes, itching, redness of your skin, high temperature, increased swelling, a fever, for possible skin infection of the area.

10. If punctures or scratches occur, wash the area with mild soap and lukewarm water, apply antibiotics, and observe for signs and symptoms of infections.

Douglass et al.'s research study on basic lymphedema self-care has been focused on meticulous skincare, which included frequent hand washing and drying of the affected area with mild soap and water. The use of medicated topical creams antibiotics for cases with skin infection, conscientious use of emollients to maintain skin integrity, and great attention to nail care, elevating the limb or area with edema while sleeping and during the daytime when possible, range of motion exercises, and the application of topical creams.

Turk J Surg. Study of 2017 emphasized the importance of proper hygiene as vital for patients with lymphedema. The use of low pH moisturizers is recommended to overcome skin cracking and drying, and for prevention of entry of microorganisms in the edematous limb.

SOME SUGGESTED SKIN CARE PRODUCTS

LOW PH SOAP: Dove, Aveeno liquid or hard soap.
LOW PH LOTION :
Eucerin, Amylactin, Lymphoderm, Vaseline cream.

WHAT IS MANUAL LYMPHATIC DRAINAGE

It is a manual therapy manipulation technique that assists the lymphatic system by aiding in varied interstitial pressures when a light pressure, popularly known as "Vodder strokes" which is applied through the skin in a unique pattern of hand movements.

Some of the known great effects and benefits of manual lymphatic drainage (MLD) include an increase in lymph production to improve fluid rerouting, increase in lymph-angiomotoricity or increase in contraction smooth muscles near the lymph collectors or vessels, increases venous return, it is soothing (most of my clients can get to the snoring stage when I do MLD to them, at times), analgesic or a pain reliever.

The main goal of this unique soft tissue manipulation is to increase fluid rerouting around the defective lymph vessels to the healthier vessels that drain to the venous system, thereby decreasing the congestion of fluid and reducing the edema.

MLD is the most sought out component of CDT by the majority of the clients that I see due to its soothing effect.

There are some general considerations prior to performing MLD. When you have one of these, we do not perform, or we perform MLD with extreme caution: cardiac edema due to heart failure, acute renal failure, active blood clots, active infection, active bleeding, and undiagnosed cancer.

Research 1: In the peer-reviewed article published at Lymphedema PDQ of the National Cancer Institute 2019, they described MLD as a type of massage technique that involves the use of a very light superficial massage with a gentle, rhythmic skin distention, with ideal pressures of approximately 30 mmHg to 45 mmHg.

Comparing to many other massage techniques, MLD is very light to the touch. The strokes often feel like a "brushing" technique.

Manual lymphedema therapy decreases congested lymph nodes by directing it to the circulatory and lymphatic system. MLD should be done first in the unaffected areas to direct the lymph away from the affected extremity.

Some pertinent points recommended by this peer review:

1. Do not perform MLD directly to any open wounds, hematomas, or areas with skin breakdown.

2. Do not perform MLD directly over tumors that are apparent on the skin surface.

3. No MLD on areas with acute deep venous thrombosis.

4. No MLD directly over soft tissue undergoing radiation therapy as the skin is sensitive.

Research 2: Another research conducted by Oliviera et al. had shown that MLD is as safe and effective as active exercises in rehabilitation after breast cancer surgery.

In their study:

- Forty-eight hours after surgery, women started the intervention (MLD or AE).

- The women assigned to the MLD group began 40-min individual MLD sessions, twice a week, for 30 days.

- The women assigned to the exercise group began 40-min group sessions (5–20 women), twice a week, for 30 days.

The study concluded that MLD is equally safe and effective as exercise in rehabilitation after breast cancer surgery. They both have the same effect on ROM, wound, lymphatic parameters for the lymphedema clients in the study up to 30 months after surgery.

WHAT IS COMPRESSION BANDAGING

Compression therapy that is effective in the treatment of lymphedema is multilayered bandaging and compression garments. These are the essential element in the long-term management of moderate and severe lymphedema. Compression therapy will aid in decreasing the swelling by reducing capillary filtration, increase LS flow, and fluid rerouting to less or noncongested areas. It will break thickened tissues from fibrosis.

Compression bandaging is required to achieve clinical and cost-effective treatment outcomes and to help patients maintain function and improve appearance. For most people with chronic lymphedema, compression therapy is the most important component of CLT.

The principles used in multi-layer compression bandaging includes:

1. Compression application is from high pressure to low pressure from distal to the proximal part of the leg or

arm (from feet to the thigh or from hands to upper arm).

2. The pressure gradient or concentration is achieved by the application of more layers at the distal portion with more overlap, using a progressively wider short stretch bandages (of a 6-cm to10-cm) from the foot up to the thigh or from hands to the upper arm.

3. Severe or stage 3 lymphedema - applying a second layer of bandages over the first to achieve higher pressure.

4. The principle of Bandaging follows the Laplace law (a pressure applied to an area of the small radius will produce higher pressure and vice versa).

During movement of the bandaged arm or leg, the resistance of the bandages creates a sufficient pressure to counteract the hydrostatic pressure of the venous system that helps in muscle pumping to reroute fluid into the lymphatic and venous vessels upwards.

When muscles are at rest and venous pressure is very low, and the pressure from bandages is also low making this tolerable for the patient.

COMMONLY USED COMPRESSION BANDAGING PRODUCTS:

ROSIDAL BANDAGE PACKAGES

COMPRILAN BANDAGEPACKAGES

UNNA BOOT (BEST FOR WEEPING EDEMA)

COMPRESSION GARMENTS

The patients with lymphedema usually transition to wearing compression garments or stockings once they reached phase II or when their legs or arms are decongested.

The compression garments have to be worn throughout the individual's life to reach the maximum amount of decongestion of the limb with lymphedema. Only a trained and certified LE therapists are allowed to give the proper judgment of the garment prescription for an individual to ensure the highest and most certain benefits of the CDT and compression garments choice and recommendations,

There are four compression levels used for LE clients. Compression lower than 20mmHg is not recommended.

Level I 20 to 30 mmHg

Level II 30 to 40 mmHg

Level III 40 to 50 mmHg

Level IV >60 mmHg

Below are some of the popular websites where compression garments you can purchase online, in-stores, or over the phone.

https://lymphedemastore.com/

http://www.juzousa.com/

https://lymphedivas.com/

https://www.lymphedemaproducts.com/

Research 1: In the study of Sugisawa et. al, they found out that "compression stockings may represent a treatment option to improve the leg pumping lymph pressure and decreases leg edema and thereby enhancing one's quality of life in healthy females with low leg pumping pressure." The following are the results of this research:

1. Wearing knee-high compression stockings for 16 weeks significantly increased the leg pumping pressure and improved quality of life in healthy female volunteers with low leg pumping pressure.

2. Comparison between two types of compression stockings with 18–29 mmHg at the ankle and 15–23 mmHg at the calf are more effective than those with pressures of 7.5–13 mmHg and 10.3–15 mmHg.

COMPRESSION PUMPS

Lymphedema compression pumps forces air through the compression sleeves with multiple chambers which houses overlapping cells. The pump pushes the air into the cells which increases lymph fluid flow to continue circulating in the lymphatic system and not become stagnant in the area of affectation.

A study conducted by Aldrich et. al, they found out that pneumatic compression therapy devices (PCTs) are considered alternative method of lymphedema compression therapy. They are popularly used in the clinics as part of lymphedema treatment, and at home as a self-management therapy. The system consists of a pump that inflates and deflates in a synchronized fashion on the garment worn over the affected area. They are generally easy to operate by the patient at home in accordance with the prescription by a licensed medical practitioner and training done by a certified lymphedema therapist.

Research 1: The Research study of Aldrich et. al in 2017, on the effectiveness of pneumatic compression therapy using pumps in lymphedema patients through "a direct visualization using a near-infrared fluorescence lymphatic imaging (NIRFLI) to see the lymphatic anatomy and its function in four subjects with primary and cancer-related lymphedema of the lower extremities. The visualization was done before, during, and after pneumatic compression therapy (PCT). The study revealed an increase in the lymphatic function, during and after PCT therapy in all subjects. However, further studies are necessary to assess the effects of PCT pressure and sequences on lymph uptake and movement."

Despite not enough good research-based evidences of the efficacy of the pump this has become widely used by many as this is an easy option to perform compared to the manual lymphatic drainage that entails thorough patient and caregiver training to follow the techniques.

What are some popular PCTs you can avail with medical provider prescription?

Flexitouch

https://www.tactilemedical.com/products/flexitouch-system/

Biocompression Systems

https://www.biocompression.com/compression-therapy-for-treatment-of-lymphedema-venous-insufficiency-and-wound-healing/

DECONGESTIVE EXERCISES

Decongestive exercises are types of exercises that is very effective for decreasing the volume of fluid in the area of swelling helping in fluid rerouting. After performing manual lymphatic drainage, compression bandaging and/or wearing the garments or compression stockings, then decongestive exercises will commence. This is considered as a very effective exercise specially during the early phase of treatment.

The exercises should be done in the following order:

Trunk, neck, shoulder, legs. Do 3 to 5 repetitions of each exercise. You may choose to do more, but it is important to follow them in order.

Important things to remember for decongestive exercises:

1.   Proper breathing techniques should be used throughout the session.

2. Exercises must be done wearing compression sleeves or bandages or stockings (except for exercises in the pool).

3. All exercises must be done twice daily for about 10-15 minutes

4. Duration of program should be slowly increased over period of time with individual's comfort.

5. Exercises must be done in slow, controlled manner. Relaxation is important in between individual types of exercises and should last at least as long as the time spent during the exercise.

6. Do not wear tight or restrictive clothing while performing the exercises.

Research 1: The research conducted by Melam et al., had shown that both clinically and statistically there was a relevant improvement in the quality of life that was observed in the complete decongestive therapy group who received remedial exercises and home program in addition to compression bandaging and manual lymphatic drainage.

The research study the exercises highlighted are the following:

    1.   Remedial exercises (consisted of diaphragmatic breathing exercises in between).

    2.   The following order was adopted for remedial exercises by a trained physical therapist.

    1) Warm up activity by active mobilization of large joints at moderate pace for 5 minutes.

    2) Shoulder girdle mobilizations (scapular retraction, protraction, depression, shoulder extension, elbow flexion and extension, wrist flexion and extension and ball squeezes).

    3) Pectorals and trapezius muscles stretching.

3. Diaphragmatic breathing. The patients were positioned seated, relaxed, placed their hands over their abdominal muscles, and took deep breaths through the nose and a prolonged expiration through mouth without any strenuous effort.

4. The one-hour home program consisted of self -
lymphatic drainage, skin care and the remedial exercises.

TABLE OF SAMPLE DECONGESTIVE EXERCISES

EXERCISES	DESCRIPTIONS
Abdominal Breathing Sit/Lying position 5-10 times	Place both hands on your belly. Inhale deeply through your nose into your belly (feel how you breathe moves your hands downward). Exhale through your mouth Perform breathing exercises as often as possible during the day
Neck Exercises Sit/Stand position 5-10 times	1. Look up and down 2. Look to the right, look to the left 3. Bring your right ear towards your right shoulder and do the same on the left side without moving your shoulders.
Shoulder Exercises Sit/stand position 5-10 times	Shoulder Rolls Rotate shoulders alternately on the right and left side. Perform shoulder rolls using both shoulders forwards and backwards Shoulder Shrugs Shrug both shoulders and inhale. Exhale while the shoulders relax

Arm/Fingers Sit/stand position 5-10 times	Place palms and fingers together Move little fingers away from each other and back together Move ring fingers away from each other and back together
Hand Sit/stand position 5-10 times	Alternate between hands, the relaxed hand rests on the leg Making a fist (Hold for 3 seconds) Open the fist (Relax hand for 3 seconds) Make a fist (rotate the wrist clock wise and counter-clockwise) Make a fist and touch it to the opposite shoulder
Arm& Hands Sit/stand position 5-10 times	Picking Oranges Stretch out arm and lean forward Make a fist and return hand to leg Climb up the Ladder Alternate between arms (continue for about 30-40 seconds) Hold arms above head Grasp rungs of imaginary ladder and "climb" as high as possible (remain seated) 1. Swimming Use breaststrokes as far as possible to the front, move arms to the side, then to the knees and to the front again 2. Push Hand to Opposite Knee (Alternate between arms)

	Place the palm of one hand on opposite knee and push down with hand, and upward with knee. Hold for five seconds
Sit/stand	Stick or Cane exercise *1.* Climb up and down the stick Hold the stick vertically between your knees with your hands Take the stick at bottom with one hand and walk up and down the stick with alternating hands *2.* Weight Lifting Hold the stick with both hands horizontally with the palms up Lift the stick up and towards your head and return to original position *3.* Wringing the Stick Hold the stick with both hands horizontally with the palms down and about one foot apart. Attempt to wring the stick moving one hand forward and the other back. (Hold for about 3-5 seconds and wring in the other direction.) *4.* Canoeing Hold the stick with both hands horizontally with the palms down and about one foot apart Start to paddle to either side with nice,

	slow and big paddle strokes.
Abdominal Breathing	Place both hands on your belly. Inhale deeply through your nose into your belly (feel how you breathe against your hands). Exhale through your mouth Perform breathing exercises as often as possible during the day
Walking	Walking is a great exercise for lymphedema of the lower extremities. Treadmill (Keep it on a low setting to avoid soreness or strain). "Remember to always try to walk with a normal gait. Do not drag the affected leg and avoid limping."
Stationary bicycle	Stationary bike or road or fitness bike keeping the setting low, speed slow as tolerated)

CHAPTER 4

THE RELATIONSHIP BETWEEN OBESITY AND LYMPHEDEMA

"OBESITY-INDUCED LYMPHEDEMA"

In this busy world of human existence, we often encounter people with various medical concerns of obesity, overweight, and on the other side of the spectrum, some suffering from underweight, and anorexia. Those who are suffering from high and low blood pressure, and stroke, diabetes, kidney problems can be averted by trudging in the normative pathway of a healthier lifestyle.

Obesity is a very familiar word in everyone's daily conversation. Consistently, we see people suffering from obesity and overweight in every corner of the society, in the community, in church, in the busy streets of the downtown area, in the grocery stores, or in the malls. It is becoming a common scenario. The effects this gives to people's mental and emotional health are also far soaring high, adding to the rate of depression and anxiety problems in the world.

Nonetheless, overweight and obesity are not uncommon in the female population. A woman's body structure is predisposed to changes during pregnancy, and the majority stalled within the post-pregnancy weight. Often it is confounded by the childbearing ability of the Venus gender. Obesity in men and women can lead to some reversible medical conditions such as diabetes, cardiovascular problems, and stroke, and other irreversible medical issues like kidney failure, and cancer depending on malignancy.

According to the Centers for Disease and Prevention, obesity is a body mass index (a healthy weight for a given height) of 30 or higher, and a BMI between 25 and 29.9 is categorized as overweight. Obesity is characterized by excess body fat.

Bodyweight is influenced by one's physiology, genetics, environment, and behavior towards nutrition and activities (Tuppo, 2015).

Weight gain is evident when the person's food intake is increased, and activities remain dormant. The more one consumes food in a sedentary lifestyle, the higher the incidence of an enormous weight gain that can readily spark obesity.

Is my body healthy and fit? Or is it unhealthy and unfit? How will I know if my body composition is in the normal range?

These are some questions we often hear when one starts to see changes in body shape and image, either getting into the slim or lean side or the opposite side of the road of being fat and obese.

So, what is body composition? According to the book of Fair 2010, a body composition is the percentage of body fat and fat-free mass or simply the lean bodyweight of an individual.

Now, "body composition wellness" is habits and practices related to the body composition, and for the physical therapist to examine or assess this, one has to monitor the patient through his/her daily activities and record this observation data.

There are five components of physical fitness: muscular strength, muscular endurance, cardiovascular endurance, flexibility, and body composition.

In my clinical experience, I do use the components of body composition wellness in the different aspects or categories of doing physical therapy complete evaluation in all my lymphedema clients. In the history taking part, using the detailed question of the patient's activity level, diet, and social, emotional, and psychological history and lifestyle are pertinent.

A comprehensive assessment of medical and surgical histories related to the integumentary system, cardiovascular and lymphatic system is crucial. Body composition examination is done by using a tape measure to gauge the size of the limb with lymphedema and the non-lymphedematous arm or leg. Taking the initial weight using the weighing scale and measuring the fat composition using a caliper, although the latter I seldom use.

It is essential to note in the assessment of the patient's past weight, the size of the limb through shoe and dress sizes, and a more vivid picture of the client's previous body size.

Research 1: A research investigation conducted by Mehrara & Greene found out that individuals with a body mass index higher than 30 had three times the risk of developing upper extremity lymphedema compared with patients with a body mass index of less than 25. There is a relationship between obesity and lymphedema. That is why it is essential to include the body composition in the history taking, systems review, tests, and measurements to have excellent clinical decision making on the approach of physical therapy and lymphedema therapy.

Research 2: In a study made by Gomes et al. (2014), they concluded that breast cancer survivors have changes in body composition and handgrip strength six months after surgery; however, the interaction between the type of surgery and its impact is unclear. Furthermore, women who developed lymphedema in this period showed more significant body composition changes, which were not enough to cause impairment in the handgrip strength.

During the systems review, I asked questions about the patient's health and nutrition, circulation problems, integumentary systems issues or past surgeries, and surgical histories involving cardiovascular, and the severance of lymphatic system and the questions on any genetic predisposition of the lymphedema and cancer treatments. Then comes incorporating health and wellness in your lymphedema therapy program to cover all aspects of the client's well-being.

One of the common challenges in assessing and managing lymphedema is measuring tissue composition, fluid amount, or amount and skin condition (body or tissue composition).

Taking care of patients with lymphedema and other obesity-related lymphedema is not an easy task because most patients have low self-esteem issues because of their body image and appearance. Most of them do not want other people to see them in their condition of having more significant or more massive and huge limbs or trunk. It is a

81

susceptible area to assess as it connotes a fragile boundary, however, with proper education on the medical issue and the hopes that the treatment approaches offer makes this sensitive issue worth fighting for in both women and men.

HOW DOES OBESITY AFFECTS LYMPHEDEMA?

Women with histories of postmastectomy are vulnerable to suffer lymphedema in the long run, especially when they fell under the obesity range.

Is there a significant relationship between obesity and lymphedema in women?

Among women with breast cancer following surgery, a greater risk of developing lymphedema of the upper extremity is 40 to 60 percent higher in women with a higher body mass index compared to women with a healthy body mass index (Zuther, 2010).

The flow chart below best represents the relationship between obesity and lymphedema (Mehrara & Greene, 2014).

82

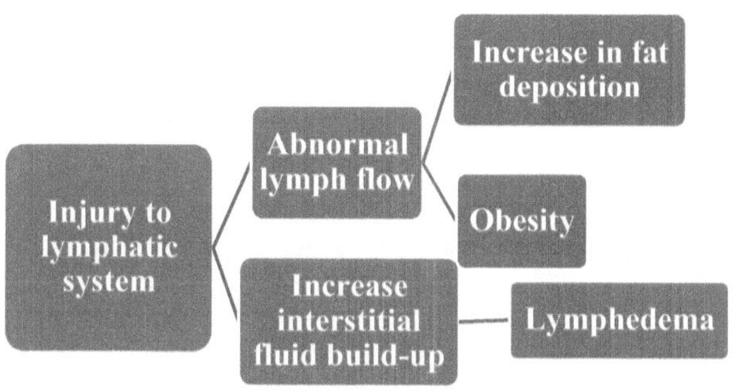

"To keep the body in good health is a duty... otherwise we shall not be able to keep our mind strong and clear." Buddha

CHAPTER 5

HEALTH AND WELLNESS FOR LYMPHEDEMA

The World Health Organization (WHO) developed what has become the most commonly referenced definition of health as, "Health is a state of complete physical, mental and social well-being and not merely the absence of disease." The definition, dated back to the 1940s, recognizes that health is more than physical health, and efforts to improve health has become comprehensive.

Wellness is defined as "the sense that one is living in a manner that permits the experience of consistent, balanced growth in the physical, spiritual, emotional, intellectual, social, and psychological dimensions of human existence

How can a health promotion initiative reverse or halt the progression of the risk factors for obesity, and obesity-related lymphedema? The cardiovascular diseases, high blood pressure, type 2 diabetes, cancers such as endometrial or cervical cancers, breast cancers in women, and other complications of obesity-related lymphedema?

The overall decrease in the quality of life among women, as well as an increasing percentage of low self-esteem leading to a rising incidence of depression, is a grim scenario.

"An ounce of prevention is worth a pound of cure." Benjamin Franklin."

Let me share my health promotion initiative program that I formatted during my doctorate program that would help avert the debilitating effects of obesity and will improve the health of women/men and the community they live in.

Weight management for obesity and obesity-related lymphedema	Description of the proposed program
Check and balance for	Assessment: Initial checking of body mass index, vital signs, and pertinent medical

members	histories.
	Programs:
	Provision of a questionnaire for individual health information, family histories and personal medical histories, lifestyles, work and hobbies.
Education and seminars. Fundraising for awareness on obesity and obesity-related lymphedema in women	Monthly training and seminars on health topics related to obesity, women's health and cancer. One yearly fundraising event to raise awareness of obesity and obesity-related lymphedema and cancer for women's health
Members: Goals, mission and vision	*Women with lymphedema empowered by a healthy lifestyle through diet and proper nutrition and an active lifestyle and wellness in both physical, emotional, psychological, intellectual, spiritual and social. * The goal is to knock-out obesity and obesity-related lymphedema in women.
Lifestyle modification and intervention	Proper diet and nutrition intervention. Regular exercises and physical activities.
Follow up yearly check and balance	End of the year tracking of BMI (Body Mass Index), health status and quality of life of all members

The above illustration of the proposed health initiative addresses the members' current health status, lifestyle and to build the group by helping each other in promoting their mission, vision, and goals for a healthier lifestyle in a busy life of women, both single and mothers with or without children.

Lifestyle modification through an intelligent life of proper diet and nutrition to get rid of obesity, and   an   active lifestyle of exercises such as brisk walking, jogging or running, Pilates, yoga, bicycling, swimming and gym activities. Tasks and events specific to their passion or interests.

The primary benefit of a healthy diet and physical activity is a reduction in the risk of obesity (HealthyPeople.gov, n.d.). Seminars and education programs on evidence-based practices related to women's health, obesity, cancer, and lymphedema. And a check and balances of members to meet their goals and working on achieving their goals for a healthier individual and community alike. The success and efficacy of the health initiative are best seen through a yearly

87

follow up of where the members stand at the end of each year on their health and well-being. A decrease in statistics in the incidence of women in the area with obesity and overweight is a fruition of the health initiative.

The data and research presented above clearly showed that there is a significant relationship between obesity and lymphedema, and the great news is, all of these debilitating risk factors of obesity and obesity-related lymphedema in women are preventable. And, with the proposed health promotion initiative for the women, healthier and well-balanced life of good health, wellness and happiness holds their future.

Health and wellness for lymphedema require consistent and dedicated effort to maintain healthy BMI and to avoid obesity if at all possible. Maintaining a balance between proper nutrition and physical fitness and exercises is the complete recipe for obtaining a healthy BMI.

It is imperative for lymphedema warriors to find their passion for what particular arena of physical activities or fitness or exercise they will be able to engage themselves in promoting a healthier way of living while continuing their journey as warriors of their lymphedema life.

To follow sound nutrition and proper dieting is the other part of the weighing scale to maintain adequate balance. The way of eating is crucial and of equal importance in doing physical fitness. Choosing the appropriate nutrition for lymphedema is crucial to make sure other comorbid conditions will be taken into consideration, for example, "follow a diabetic diet for people with diabetes, cardiac diet for those with heart conditions, and kidney diet for people with kidney diseases."

CHAPTER 6

EXERCISES FOR LYMPHEDEMA

"Health is a state of complete physical, mental and social well-being, and not merely the absence of disease or infirmity".
W.H.O.

One of the components of lymphedema therapy is exercise, which is better known as decongestive exercises.

The type of exercise that is deemed best for lymphedema is a light or subtle range of motion, strengthening, and stretching exercises in which you move the edematous arms or legs to enhance the increase in lymph fluid flow. Deep breathing exercises help wake up the deeper lymphatic vessels and improved drainage of lymph fluid to the venous system. It is important to note that the activities designed for the clients with lymphedema are never strenuous but are focused on gentle muscle contraction of the affected areas.

One of the simplest explanations for clients with regard to what happens in lymphedema during decongestive exercises and why is it necessary to perform these exercises is by giving them a scenario. In my practice I do the imagination story. "I would like you to imagine looking at the water of a very calm river, we know that it is flowing, but we can't see them in our naked eye. Placing a force on the water, such as paddling the water when you are riding your kayak or canoe, or just by even using your hands and splashing the water in a direction you wanted, you will see the water in the river flows. The mechanism describes what happens with exercise in lymphedema. Accordingly, physiology showed that muscle contraction through exercises will increase the fluid drainage more than 50%, and in addition to the compression from either the bandages or the garments one wears increasing the lymph flow more.

A certified lymphedema therapist can teach and carry out the most appropriate exercises for lymphedema clients.

What are some of the evidenced-based research that says about exercises in lymphedema?

Research 1:

91

Guatam AP et al research.

In the past, exercises for clients with lymphedema were once considered to be unsafe. A new 8-week home-based exercise research was conducted on postmastectomy patients, which has revealed an improvement in the limb/limbs affected by decreasing both its size and circumference and overall improving the person's quality of life. Increase in overall circulation that aids in removing lymph fluid in the areas affected, and with exercise, it enhances total weight loss, thereby decreasing swelling of the limbs.

Research 2:
Wanchai A, Armer JM research

A second study in using heavy resistance exercises for the upper body revealed that training was effective in improving strength, the endurance of the muscles, and the client's overall quality of life. However, swelling and severity remain the same. In conclusion, the researchers said that resistance training was found to be safe in patients with lymphedema.

92

Research 3:

Nelson NL systematic review research.

Another investigation in the form of a systematic review of existing literature found out that resistance exercise does not exacerbate breast cancer-related lymphedema. And that both aerobic and strength training exercise during and after cancer treatment is safe to be prescribed that enhances the range of motion, muscular strength of affected areas and improves overall fitness and quality of life. And should be administered by a physical therapist, occupational therapist, or cancer or a lymphedema therapist that had the proper training.

Research 4:

Şener, H. Ö et, al, 2017 research on clinical Pilates and lymphedema.

A more recent study on the effects of Clinical Pilates Exercises on lymphedema patients', was found out that clinical Pilates exercises had a positive impact on the amount of lymphedema, functional status, grip strength, and quality of life of patients with lymphedema.

It was considered to be a good exercise regimen and can be adapted as a lifestyle modification type of exercise.

Other positive effects of clinical Pilates exercises on the patient with breast cancer who developed lymphedema after their treatment includes improved functionality, mood, and quality of life. In this study, clients in both the clinical Pilates and control group were recommended to wear pressure garments on the arm with lymphedema during the treatment sessions.

Muscle contraction during exercises under adequate compression of the affected limb is effective for lymphedema. When the edematous limb is compressed on the skin surface, this causes an increase in the pumping muscular movement in the subcutaneous tissue and directly increases the massaging effects through intermittent increases in the tissue pressure, which in turn decreases the leakage of fluid from capillaries thereby reducing edema. However, excessive or strenuous exercise may cause inflammation and should be avoided.

"You beat cancer by how you live, why you live, and in the manner in which you live."
Anonymous

CHAPTER 7

DIET AND NUTRITION FOR LYMPHEDEMA

There is no specific diet for lymphedema.

We learned in Chapter 3 that there is a direct relationship between obesity and lymphedema risk in some primary or secondary type. Therefore, it is essential to maintain a healthy BMI (body mass index) or average weight. Excessive weight increases the workload of the lymphatic systems to perform fluid drainage, thereby decreasing its ability to decongest the area. Therefore, proper weight management will positively affect lymphedema.

The best nutritional approach in the management of lymphedema is to follow a balanced diet, coupled with physical fitness and exercises, and wellness to promote healthy body mass index.

The nutrition and diet for lymphedema are comorbidity specific. When one has diabetes, hypertension, cancer, kidney disease, heart failure, and other health issues, critical food, or nutrition is specific to the diet suggestion of each illness. The idea is a balanced diet and keeping the weight at its normal range. It is a choice of following either a low-fat diet, a high healthy fat diet, a low-carb diet, diabetic or sugar-free, gluten-free diet and low salt or healthy heart diet, and vegan or vegetarian diet.

There are plenty of choices out there, as long as weight is controlled, and fluid reduction is also maintained, the type of diet one chooses is a comorbid-medical condition specific.

Studies indicate that obesity does have an influence on lymph fluid levels and extremity volume. Obesity and overweight often worsen the symptoms associated with lymphedema; nutrition balanced, and appropriate portion diet contributes to reducing the risk factors associated with lymphedema.

A balanced healthy diet, including whole grains, fish, fruits, and vegetables, and avoiding fatty foods will

97

significantly assist in achieving and maintaining a healthy weight without restricting the intake of essential nutrients and vitamins. Some diets which limiting certain food groups and nutrients are not advisable. There is a common misconception that lymphedema may be positively affected by restricting protein intake. Although lymphedema is defined as an accumulation of water and protein in the tissues, it is essential to understand that lymphedema cannot be reduced by the limitation of protein ingestion, which can even be potentially dangerous. It is also important not to limit fluid intake in an attempt to reduce the swelling. Proper hydration (water) is essential for primary cell function and especially crucial before and after lymphedema treatment to assist the body in eliminating waste.

Some suggested ways of eating that would maintain proper nutrition, weight control, and normal BMI.

The low carb, moderate, and high good fat diet (i.e., Ketogenic diet, Paleo diet), the intermittent fasting diet, and your blood type diet are some of the popular diet fads in the 20th century.

The ketogenic diet is mainly consisting of high-fats (good fats), moderate-proteins, and very-low-carbohydrates. The percentages of the macronutrients that are being strictly followed by people doing this diet are the following: approximately 55% to 60% fat, 30% to 35% protein, and 5% to 10% carbohydrates. These percentages are based on a 2000 kcal per day diet, and carbohydrates amount up to 20 to 50 g per day.

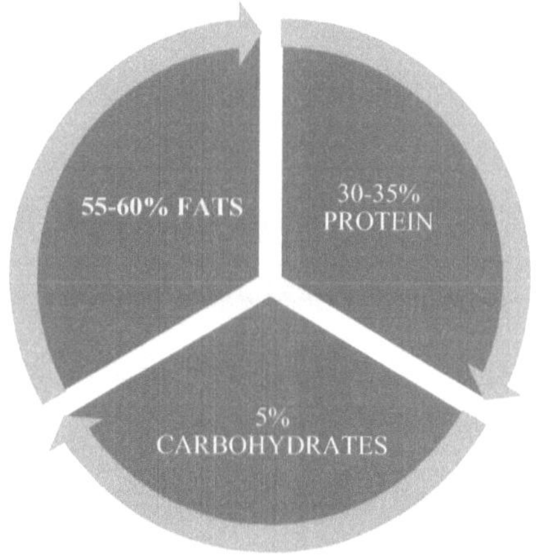

In a ketogenic diet, the body tissues are deprived of carbohydrates which are the prime source of its energy production. The insulin production is significantly reduced, when the carbohydrates is decreased by 50 mg per day or less.

When the body's secretion of carbohydrates is lowered, there are two metabolic processes that come into action (1) gluconeogenesis is the endogenous production of glucose in the body, especially in the liver primarily from lactic acid, glycerol, and the amino acids alanine and glutamine. (2) Ketogenesis due to low blood glucose feedback, the stimulus for insulin secretion is also low, which sharply reduces the stimulus for fat and glucose storage.

When the availability of glucose are decreased greatly, the endogenous production of glucose is not able to keep up with the needs of the body, and ketogenesis starts to provide an alternate source of energy in the form of ketone bodies. Ketone bodies replace glucose as a primary source of energy. A "nutritional ketosis" occurs as long as the body is deprived of carbohydrates, the metabolism remains in the ketotic state. It is considered quite safe, as ketone bodies are produced in small amount without any alterations in blood pH. It imperatively differs from ketoacidosis, which is a life-threatening condition where ketone bodies are produced in enormous concentrations, altering blood ph to an acidotic state.

Paleolithic or Paleo diet is a way of eating which mimics the early human existence way of eating like our hunter-gatherer ancestors thousands to millions of years ago. People eat on what their environment provides them. It could be low carb with high animal foods or could be high carb with plenty of plant-based foods. The main thought of this type of diet is to consume whole foods and avoiding processed foods.

The diet has low carbohydrate and lean protein of 30 to 35% daily caloric intake, fiber diet from non-cereal, plant-based, and is up to 45 to 100 g daily. Like the ketogenic diet, the body tissues are deprived of carbohydrates, which are the prime source of its energy production. Insulin production is significantly reduced when the carbohydrates are reduced by 50 mg per day or less.

When the body's secretion of carbohydrates is reduced or lowered, there are two metabolic processes that happens, gluconeogenesis is the endogenous production of glucose in the body, especially in the liver primarily from lactic acid, glycerol, and the amino acids alanine and glutamine.

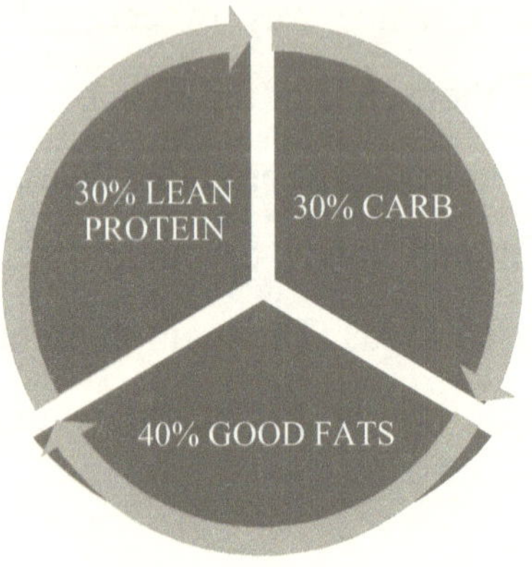

The diet has excellent effects on metabolic syndrome, blood pressure, glucose tolerance, insulin secretion, lipid profiles, and cardiovascular risk factors.

In an evidenced research of short-term randomized controlled trials, have found effects of weight loss, and improved glycemia and adipocytokine profiles, and benefits of managing diabetes in people on the paleo diet.

The Blood -Type diet, a very interesting way of eating, and according to this diet one is advised to eat in accord to their ABO blood group to improve their health and decrease risk of chronic illnesses.

According to the author of the book, ''Eat Right For Your Type'' published in 1996 by P.J. D'Adamo, there is a link between ABO blood group and diet.

The diet claims that:

- The blood-type O is known as the ancestral blood group in humans, with their choice of diet follows the high animal protein diets typical of the hunter-gatherer age.

- The type A group are the vegetarians as this blood group was believed to have existed when humans settled down into agrarian civilization.

- Individuals with blood group B will benefit from consumption of dairy products because this blood group was believed to originate in nomadic tribes.

- Individuals with an AB blood group are believed to benefit from a diet that is intermediate to those proposed for group A and group B.

- The diet also recommends that lectins, which are sugar-binding proteins found in some foods, could cause agglutination if they are not compatible with an individual's ABO blood group.

In the research study of Wang et. al, they stated that the association between blood type-based dietary patterns and health outcomes has not been examined. The objective of their study was to determine the association between 'blood-type' diets and biomarkers of cardiometabolic health and whether an individual's ABO genotype modifies any associations. Adherence to certain 'Blood-Type' diets is associated with favorable effects on some cardiometabolic risk factors, but these associations were independent of an individual's ABO genotype, so the findings do not support the 'Blood-Type' diet hypothesis.

With scarcity of scientific evidence on nutrition or diet for people with lymphedema, one is left to decide what is best nutrition they can consume to make sure that the swelling and issues with inflammation brought about by the lymphatic system problem. A great guidance from a dietician, medical doctors and a certified lymphedema therapist would be the safest route to take at this time that there is no enough scientific evidence for a specific diet for this condition. At the end of the day, your decision to stay healthy depends on great mindset coupled with good mentors or coaches like your doctors, dieticians or lymphedema therapists.

In the research study conducted by Borman, 2018, it was found out that there is no special diet in the management of lymphedema. However, in lymphocytic enteropathy or celiac disease (*a genetic, autoimmune condition in which eating gluten "a protein found in wheat, rye and barley" causes damage to the small intestine)*, food has an impact just in this particular condition.

Borman's research showed that:

1. A healthy and well-balanced diet is needed for general health.

2. Avoid decreasing or reducing fluid intake or low-protein diets.

3. There is a higher risk of lymphedema complications among women who were obese or with body mass index >30 kg/m2.

105

4. Weight gain after breast cancer has also been suggested as a risk factor in BCRL.

5. Weight loss interventions produced a significant reduction in upper extremity lymphedema volume in patients with BCRL.

6. Patients are advised to maintain a healthy BMI and weight control, as obesity is associated with inflammation and worsening of lymphedema.

SAMPLE DIET PLANS

DIET	BREAKFAST	LUNCH	DINNER
KETO	Almond/Coco flour homemade pancake 2 eggs fried/boiled 2 to 3 slices of bacon/sausage Bulletproof coffee/Tea/Water Green salad	Cauliflower fried rice Baked wild salmon with asparagus Water Strawberry Blueberry fruits	Angus steak cooked with Ghee butter Sautéed Brussels sprouts Water
INTERMITTENT FASTING 16:8	11AM -2PM scrambled eggs with	5-7PM Pork	

| | avocado , tomatoes & mushrooms

2 -3 sausages or slices of bacon
2 pieces small almond chocolate

waffle

Bulletproof coffee or tea, glass of water | tenderloin with Butternut squash & zucchini

1 small piece Boiled sweet potato

A glass of Ice water
3 scoops of low carb strawberry ice cream | |
| **PALEO DIET** | Fried broccoli in coconut oil with toasted almonds and poached egg

1 cup of coffee with no sugar | Mixed salad with tuna
Iced green tea

Dark chocolate | Beef stir fry with mixed pepper using coconut oil to fry
A glass of red wine |

For recipes please refer to specific diet recipe books. I have placed a link in the lymphedema products chapter. I personally follow the ketogenic and intermittent fasting diet as these types works well for my lifestyle. Again, in summary, one has to find his or her diet and nutrition that are specific to one's comorbid conditions and at the same time make sure these will be in conformation with your well-being not starving yourself to lose the extra pounds but to eat the right meal plans that enhances your energy and at the same time places you in the normal body mass index category as much as possible.

FOOD PYRAMID SAMPLE

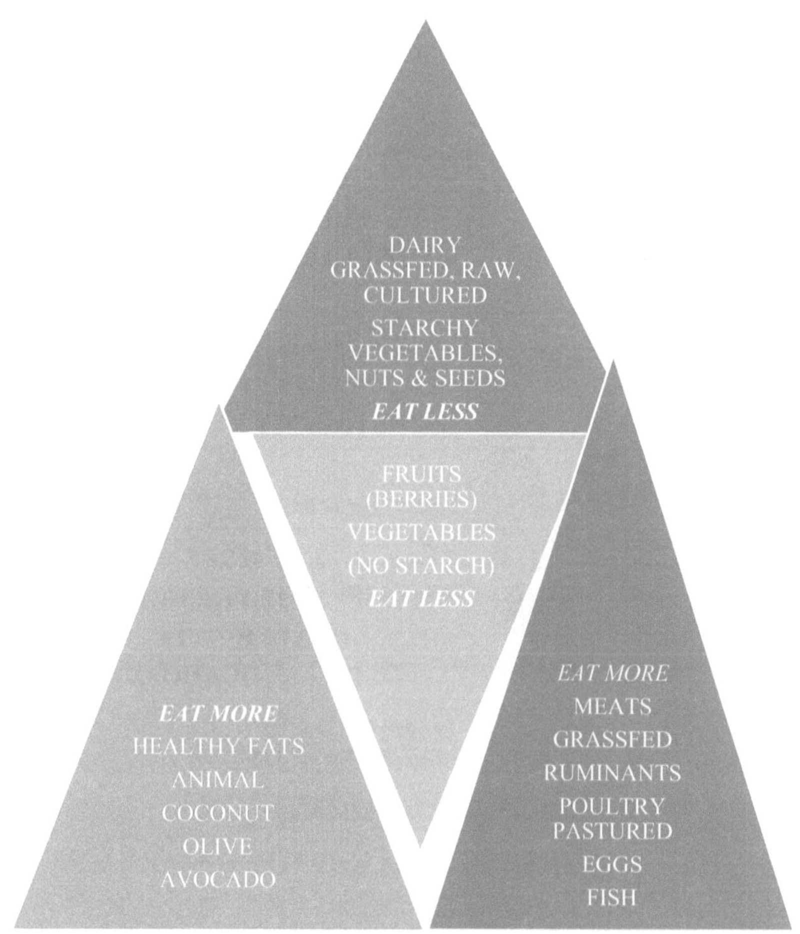

PALEO FOOD PYRMAID

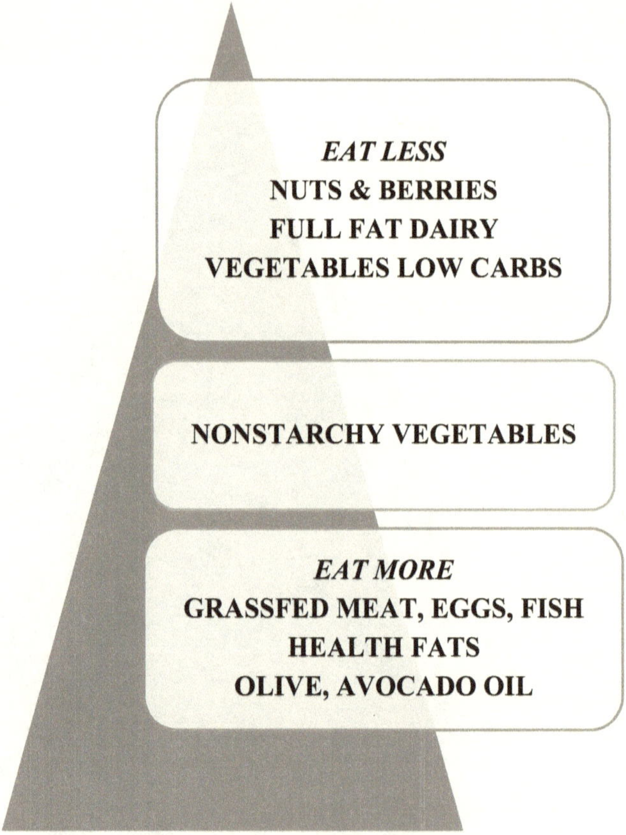

EAT LESS
NUTS & BERRIES
FULL FAT DAIRY
VEGETABLES LOW CARBS

NONSTARCHY VEGETABLES

EAT MORE
GRASSFED MEAT, EGGS, FISH
HEALTH FATS
OLIVE, AVOCADO OIL

KETOGENIC DIET PYRAMID

CHAPTER 8

SELF MANAGEMENT OF LYMPHEDEMA

The second phase of complete decongestive therapy (CDT) for the treatment of lymphedema is the self-management phase, also known as the reductive phase, which begins when a maximum reduction or utmost decrease in size of the leg or arm is achieved.

The reductive phase involves 24-hour, multilayer compression bandaging, daily manual lymphatic drainage, remedial exercises, and skincare under the care of a certified lymphedema therapist.

In this stage, it is crucial that one has the ability to manage the signs and symptoms of complications, self-treatment, physical and psychosocial side effects, and lifestyle changes in living with this chronic issue.

111

MAINTENANCE PHASE

Daily compression.

A daytime custom-made or standard garment and nighttime bandages or garment.

Compression therapy (self-managed) Multilayer, short-stretch bandages, worn 24 h/d (reductive) or during nighttime (maintenance)

Custom-made, flat-knit compression garment (arm sleeve and glove), worn during daytime (maintenance).

Self MLD

Self-massage, self- manual lymphatic drainage

*Exercise*s

Decongestive exercises, walking, any aerobics or strengthening exercises of choice, refer to Chapter on exercises.

112

Daily Exercise Deep breathing or Decongestive exercises

Proper skin care

a. Daily washing with mild soap and lukewarm water

b. Skin care careful hygiene and application of low-pH moisturizer

c. Daily Regular skin inspection for cracks, wounds, or infections

SAMPLE DAILY SELF MANUAL LYMPHATIC DRAINAGE

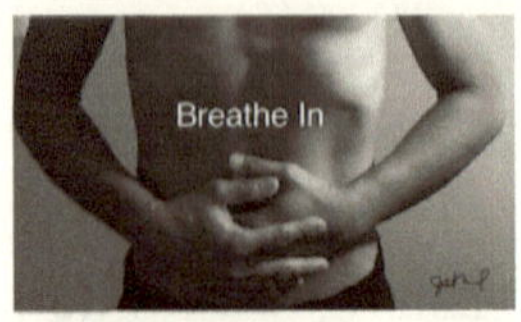

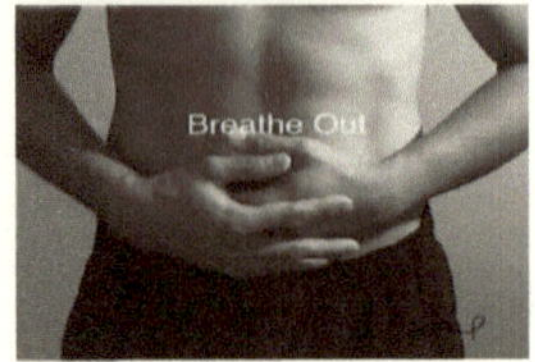

Position #1 Deep breathing. All Self MLD begins with Deep breathing to stimulate the lymphatic system of the whole body.

Perform five times. Breathe in and stomach expands. Breathe out and stomach flattens. Take a short rest in between breathes to avoid dizziness.

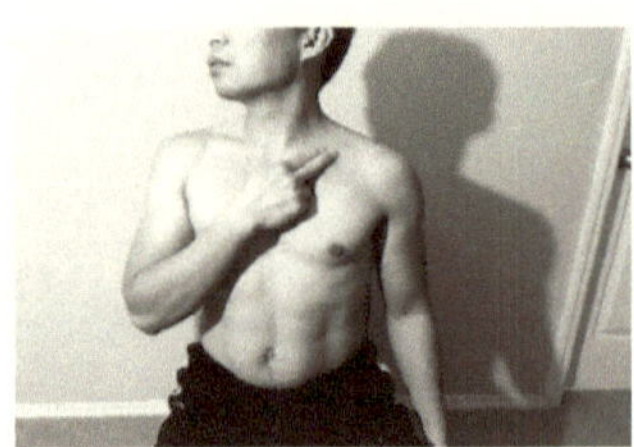

POSITION #2. Stretch & Release skin front/anterior part of the neck. Place your 2nd and 3rd fingers on either side of your neck above the collarbone. Massage down and inward towards the collarbone and gently stretch the skin with no pain and then let go of the stretch skin.

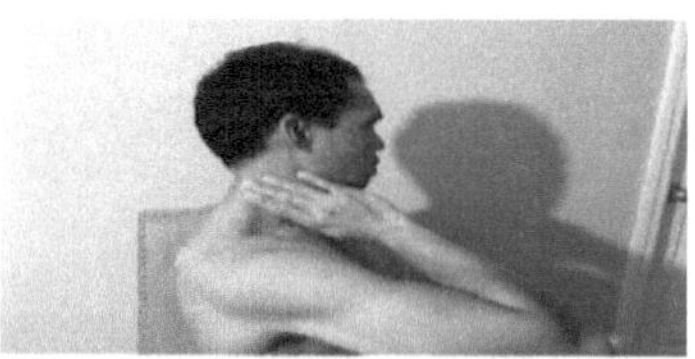

Position #3. Stretch and release at the side of the neck. Place your hands flat on the side of your neck. Gently stretch the skin away from your face downward direction, and then release. Gentle stretch of your neck and side of face in a slow and gentle manner. Repeat 10 times.

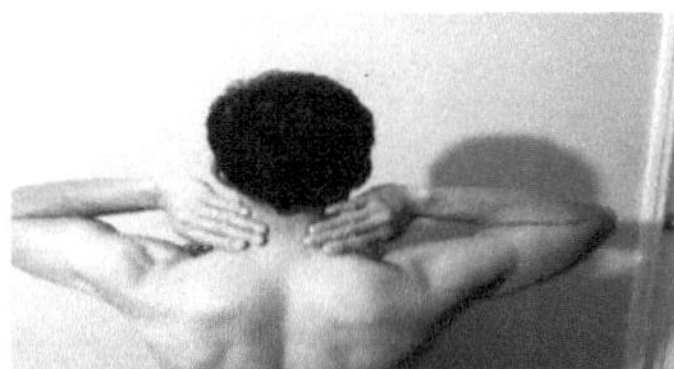

Position #4. Stretch and release the skin on the back of neck. Place the palms of your hands on the back of your neck, just below your hairline. Stretch your skin towards the spine in a downward direction and repeat 10 times.

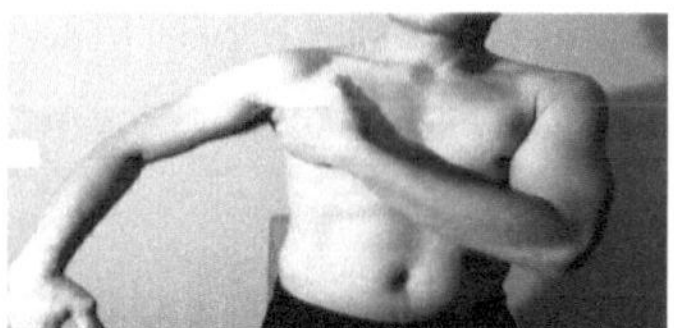

Position #5. Preparing the underarm lymph nodes/MLD for chest area. Place palm in your armpit on the affected side. Gently pull in and towards your body, and then release. Repeat 10-15 times. Repeat on the other armpit 10-15 times.

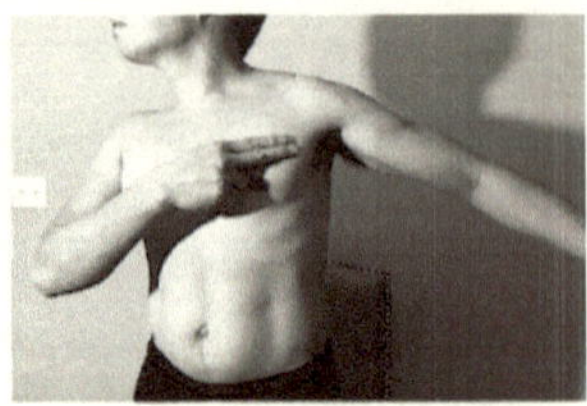

POSITION # 6. Scar tissue massage. (You can start at 3 weeks post-surgery). Move up & down in a zigzag pattern along the scar line, applying firm gentle pressure while moving along and gently lifting the skin on the scar line. Repeat 5 to 6 times.

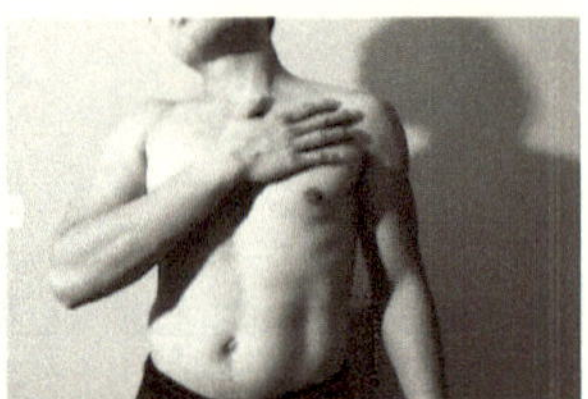

POSITION #7. Stretch & Release skin from upper chest towards the neck to move fluid up to the neck. Post-mastectomy, place hand above the scar, gently stretch the skin as far and then release. Repeat 10-15 times. Post-lumpectomy Place hand on your chest above your breast.

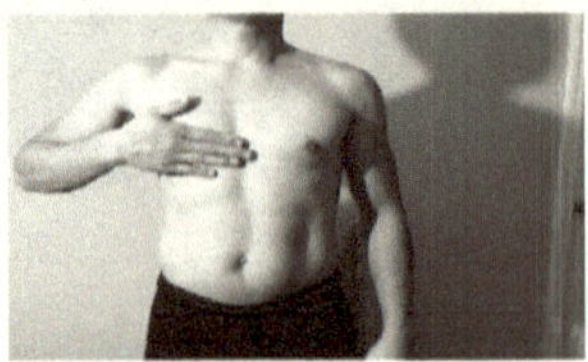

Position # 8. Preparing your chest. Place hand by your underarm on the affected side. Gently stretch & release using very small strokes across the chest towards the good side. Repeat 10-15 times.

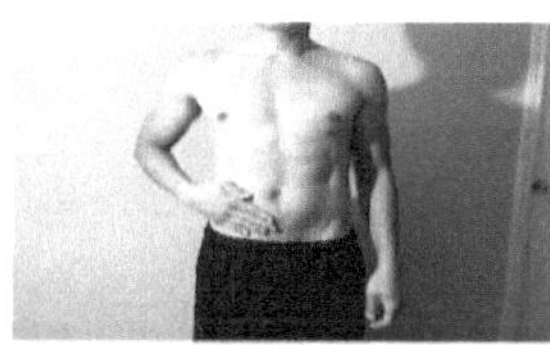

Position # 9. Preparing your groin. Stationary circles or gentle stretch & release on the affected side in an upward towards the belly button direction. Hand is steady in one spot just above the groin. Repeat 10-15 times.

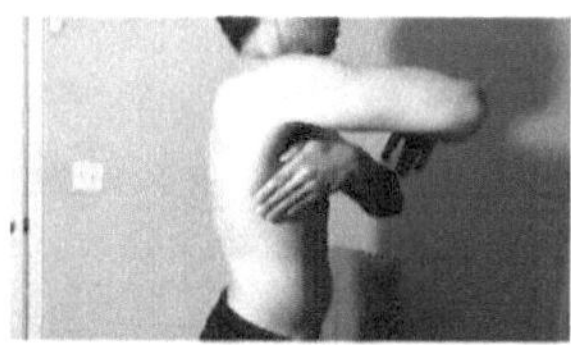

Position #10. Stretch & Release/stationary circles of the skin in a downward direction from the armpit of the affected side to the groin repeat 10-15 times.

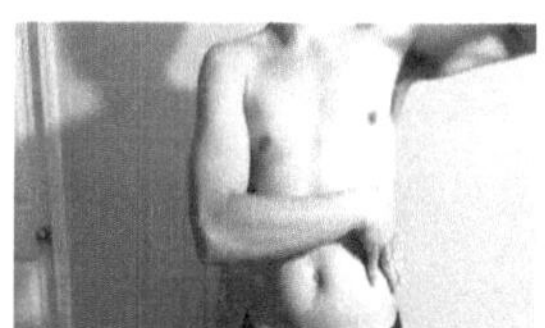

Position #11. Stretch & release of the skin from chest to your groin on the affected side

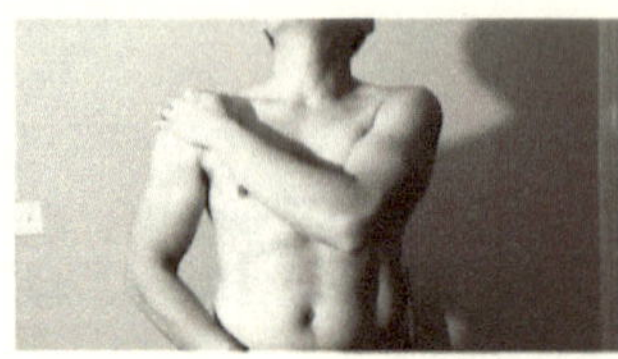

Position #12. Stretch & Release of the skin of the upper arm to the neck.

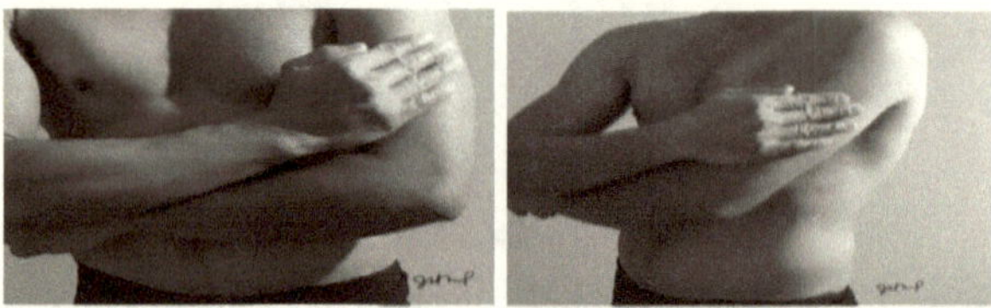

Position #13. Stretch & release from the elbow towards the shoulder.

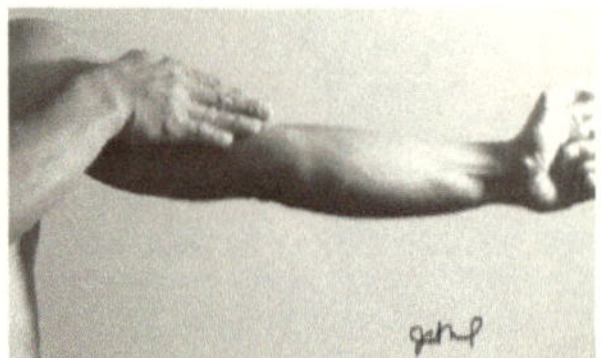

Position #14. Stretch and release /stationary circles of the skin of the arm from the inner side to the outer side.

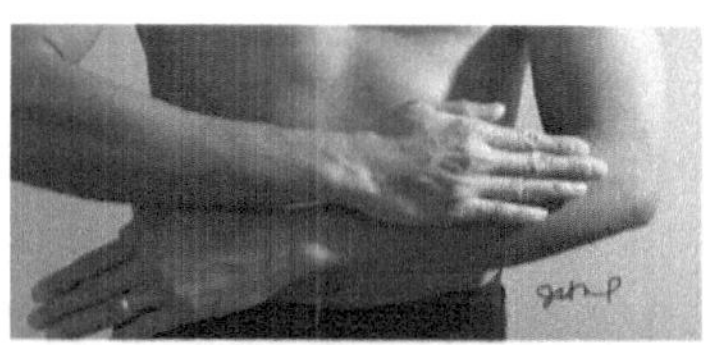

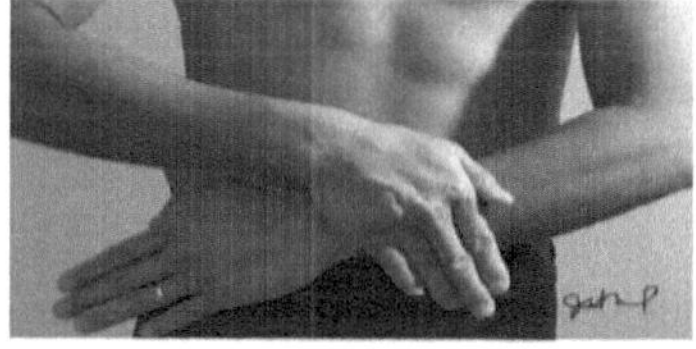

Position # 15. Stationary circles (stretch skin & release) from the wrist to the elbow, 5 to 7 times.

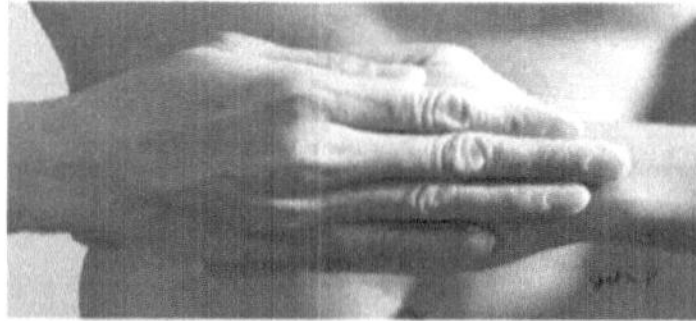

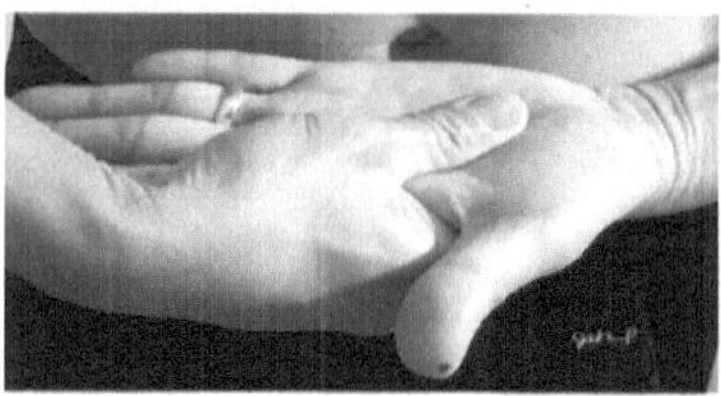

Position # 16. Stretch And release of skin of back of the hand and stretch and release of the skin of the palm of the hand. Repeat 5 to 10 times

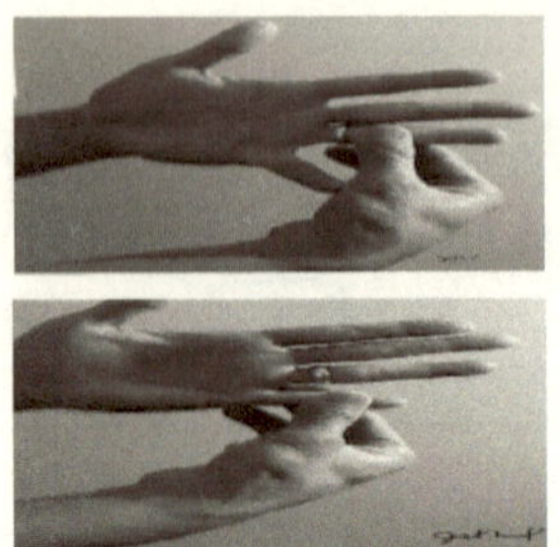

Position # 17. Stretch & release of fingers starting from little finger to the thumb from distal to proximal.

LOWER BODY SELF MLD

POSITION #1. FOR DEEP BREATHING.

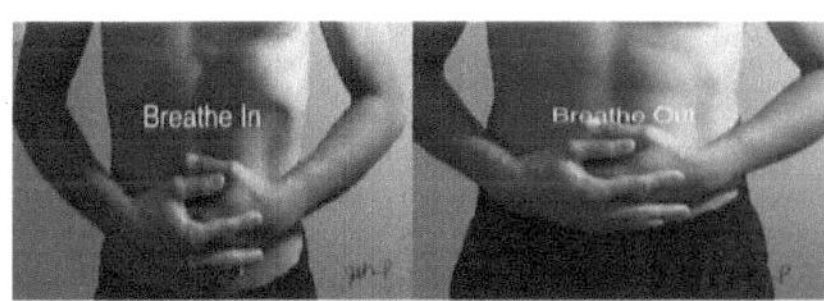

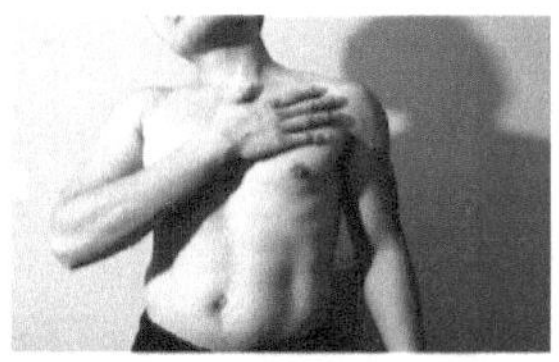

POSITION # 2. STATIONARY CIRLES from the collarbone to the neck on both sides

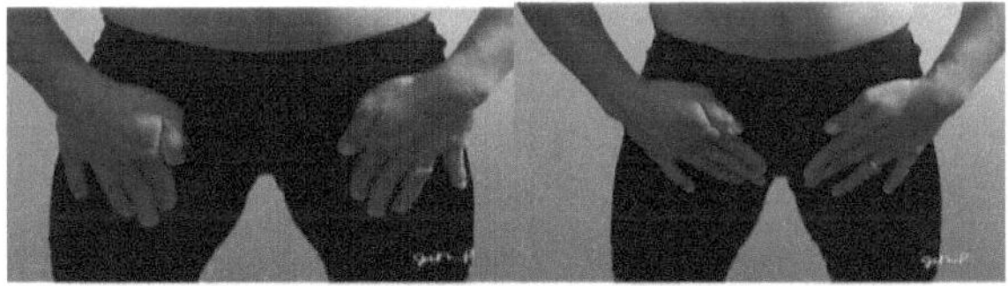

POSITION # 3. Stationary Circles from the upper inner thigh towards the groin.

121

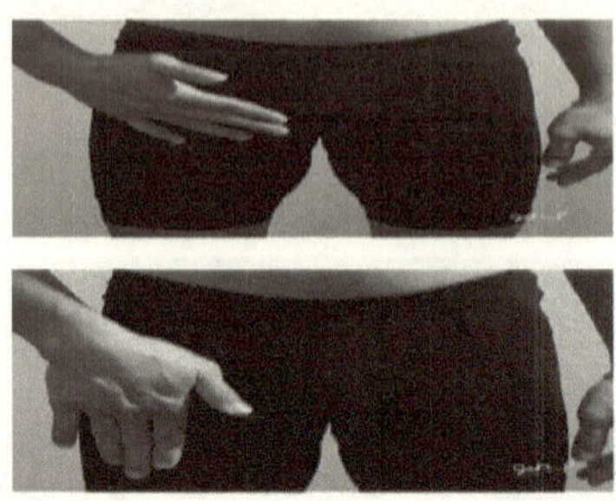

Position #4. Stationary circles from the lateral side of the thigh towards the inner side, 5 to 7 times.

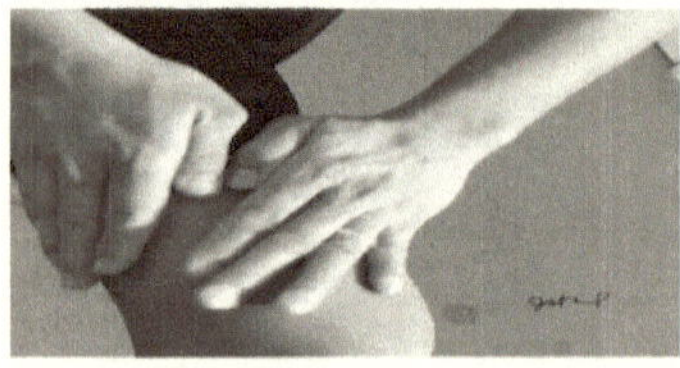

Position #5. Stationary circles from the outer thigh to the inner thigh, 5 to 7 times

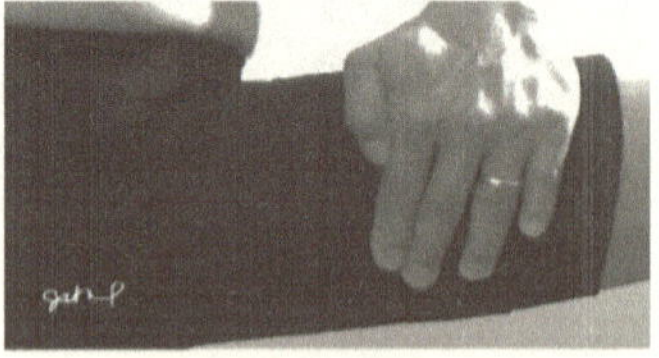

Position # 6. Stationary circles of the lateral side of the thigh from knee to the hips

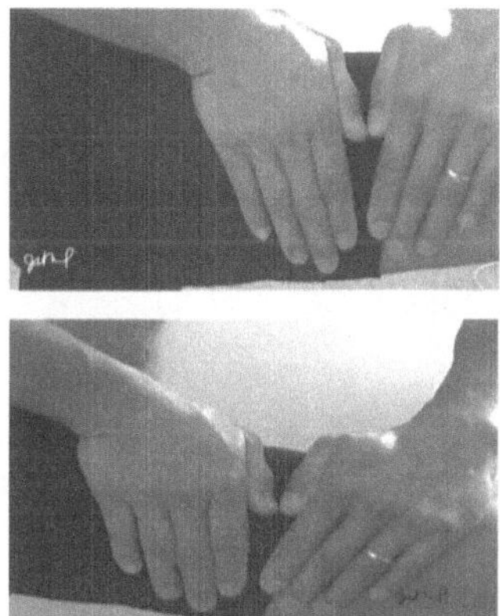

Position #7. Stretch & Release of the skin of the lateral thigh form the knee up to the hip area, 5 to 7 times

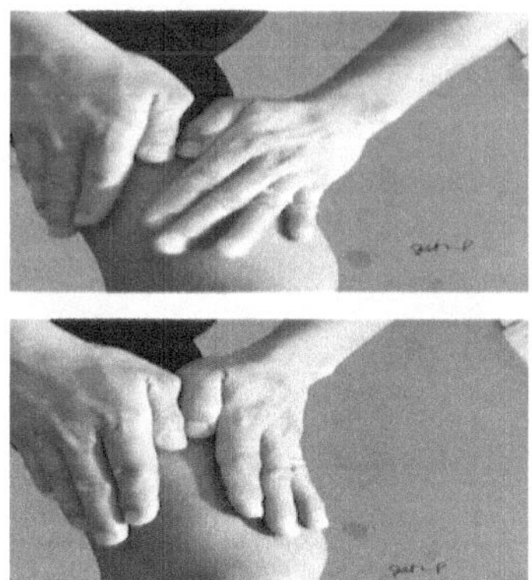

Position #8. Stretch & Release of the skin of the thigh from the inner side to the outer side.

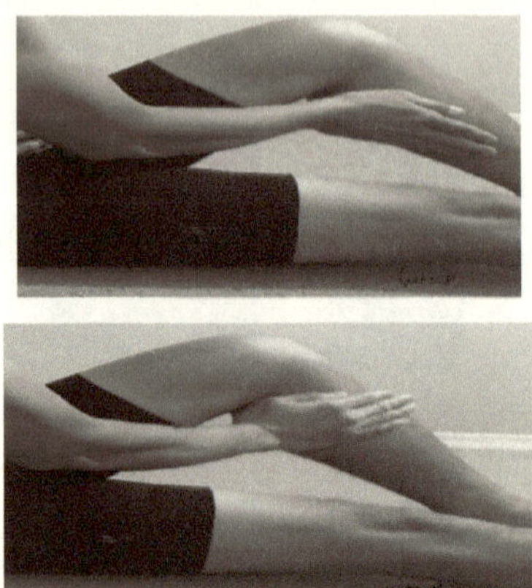

Position #9. Stretch and release of the skin of lower leg from inner to the outer side, 5 to 7 times.

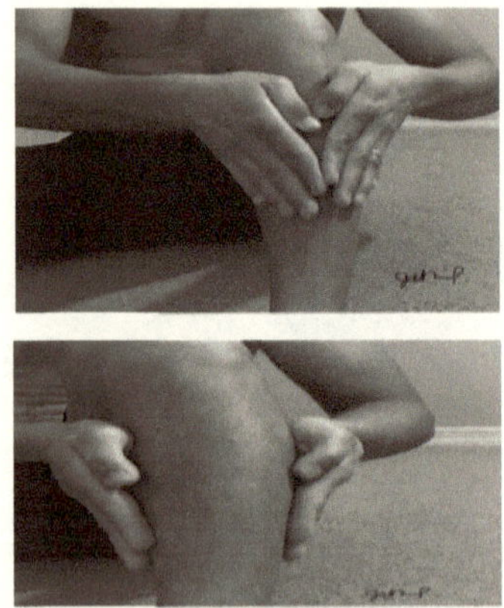

Position#10. Stretch & release of the skin from the sides to the front of the leg, 5 to 7 times.

NECK MANUAL LYMPHATIC DRAINAGE

DEEP BREATHING 5 TIMES.

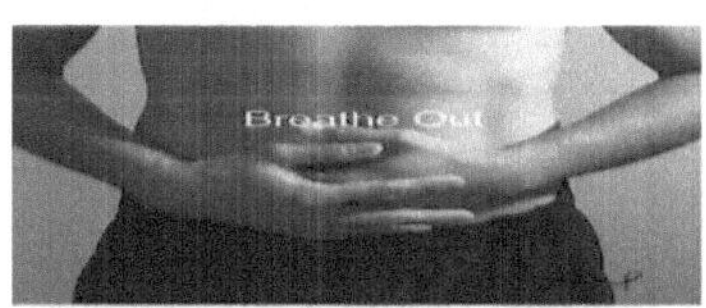

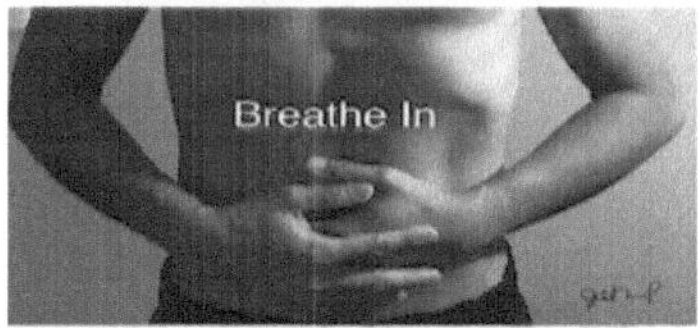

Take a short rest in between breathes to avoid dizziness.

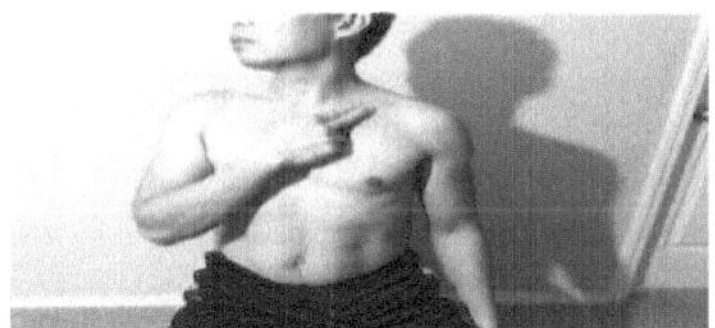

STRETCH & RELEASE OF ANTERIOR NECK SKIN

Place your 2nd and 3rd fingers on either side of your neck above the collarbone. Massage down and inward towards the collarbone and gently stretch the skin with no pain and then let go of the stretch skin. "Form a 2 letter J's, with this technique"

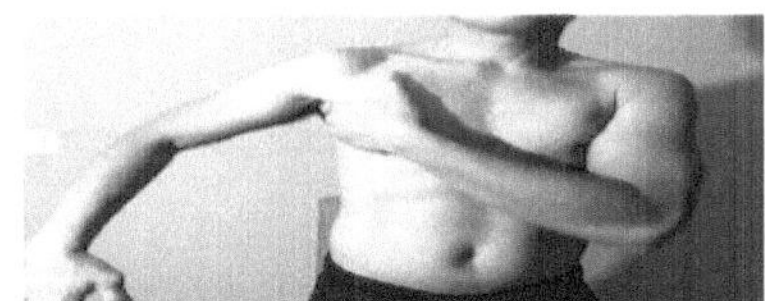

Preparing the underarm lymph nodes

Place palm in your armpit. Gently pull in and towards your body, and then release. Repeat 10-15 times. Repeat on the other armpit 10-15 times.

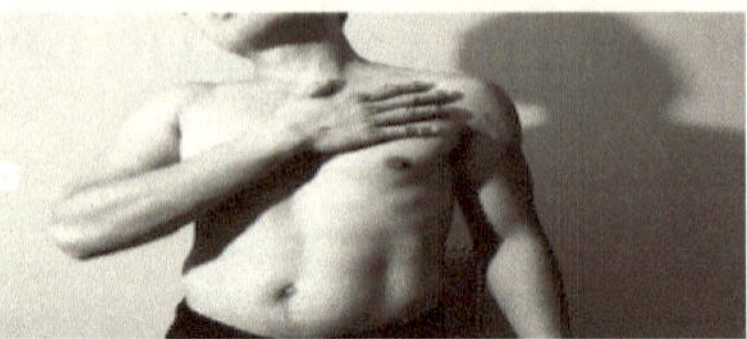

Stretch and release skin from breast area towards the armpit. Place your hand over the collarbone. Gently stretch the skin down your chest and towards the armpit forming half circles. Let go of the skin. Repeat 15 times.

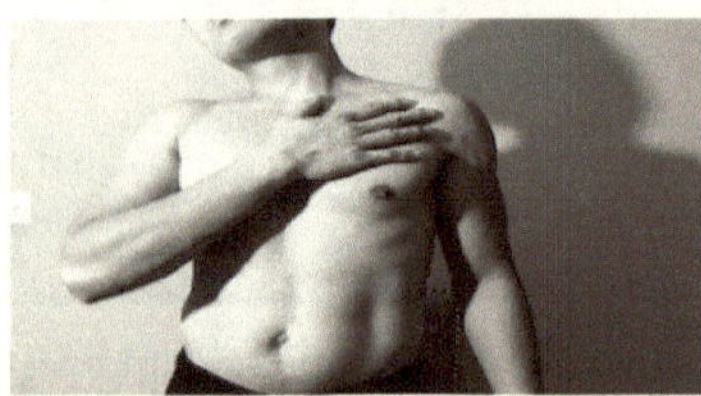

Stretch and release of the skin from the front of neck towards the chest. Place your hand over the swelling at the front of your neck. Gently stretch the skin towards the collarbone. Then let go of the skin. Repeat

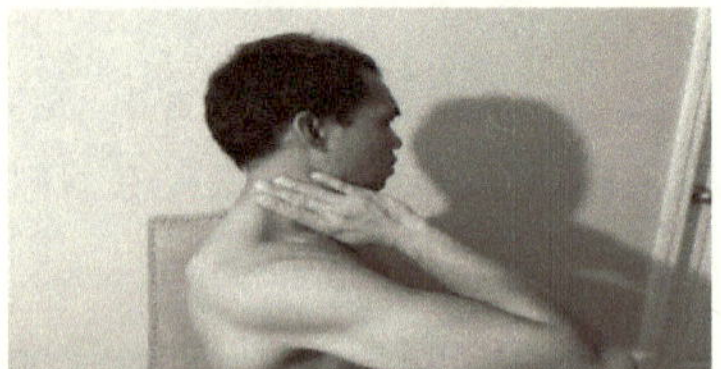

Stretch and release at the side of the neck. Place your hands flat on the side of your neck. Gently stretch the skin away from your face downward direction, and then release.

Gentle stretch of your neck and side of face in a slow and gentle manner. Repeat 10 times.

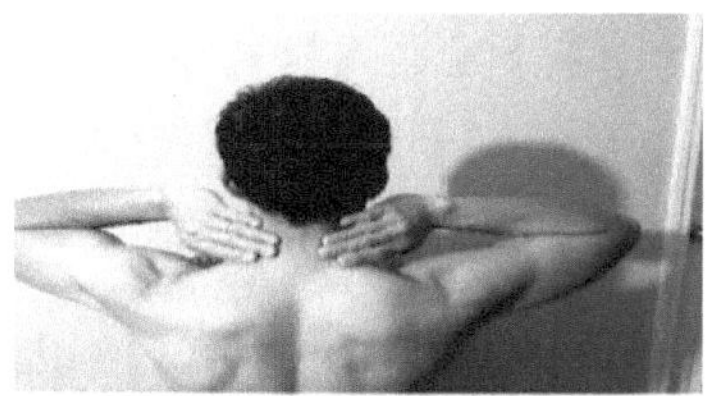

Stretch and release the skin on the back of neck.

Place the palms of your hands on the back of your neck, just below your hairline.

Stretch your skin towards the spine in a downward direction and repeat 10 times.

DAILY SKIN CARE FOR YOUR LYMPHEDEMA

Careful and thorough daily skin checks. (Look for signs of redness, abrasions, tears, scratches or cuts, and treat them accordingly. Signs of cellulitis seek medical attention ASAP for proper medications).

Daily skin cleansing. Wash swollen area thoroughly, and paying extra attention to the skin folds, webs in between toes and fingers with soap and lukewarm water. Then completely dry your skin by patting and not rubbing with clean towels or cloth.

Use Soap/soap substitute: Aqueous cream emulsifying ointment, E45 wash. Bath oils: Aveeno, E45 bath oil, oilatum.

Moisturize your skin daily. Regular nighttime moisturizing of the affected areas with proper emollients to rehydrate the skin and make it smooth.

Examples of emollients: Creams, lotions, Vaseline, Aveeno, Neutrogena, Eucerin, Lymphoderm, petroleum jelly, coconut oil.

DAILY COMPRESSION VELCRO WRAP BANDAGING

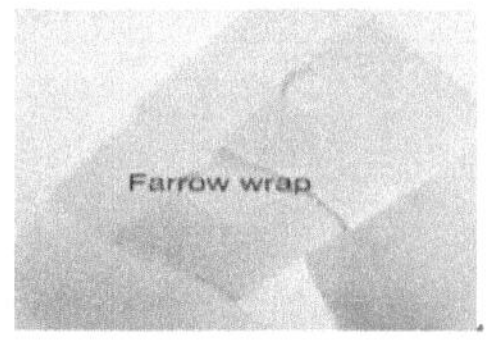

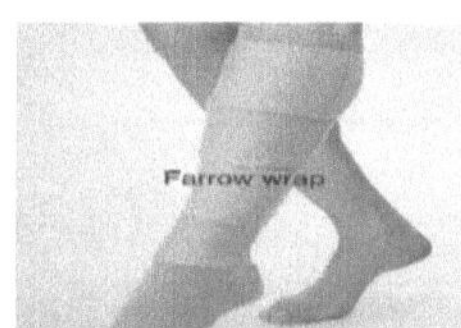

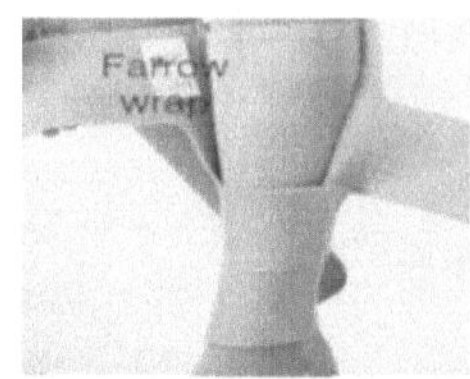

DAILY COMPRESSION LEG OR ARM PUMP

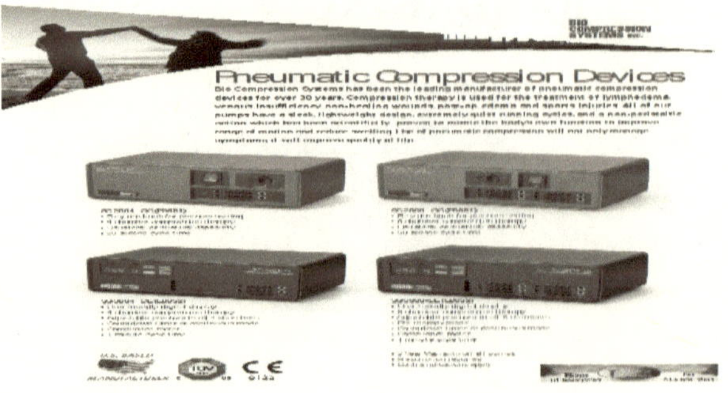

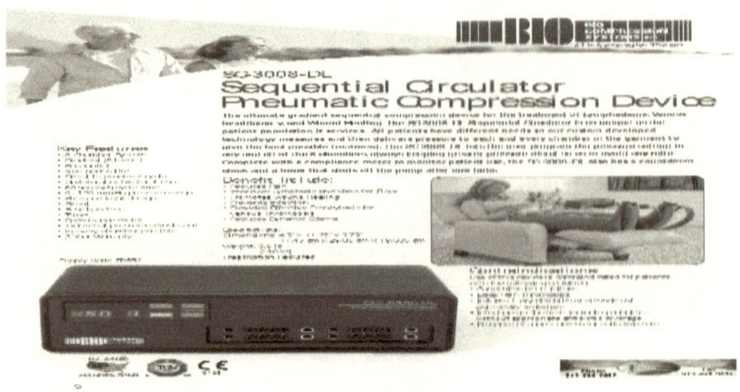

Above picture is a sample leg compression pump

SAMPLE DECONGESTIVE EXERCISES

DEEP BREATHING EXERCISES

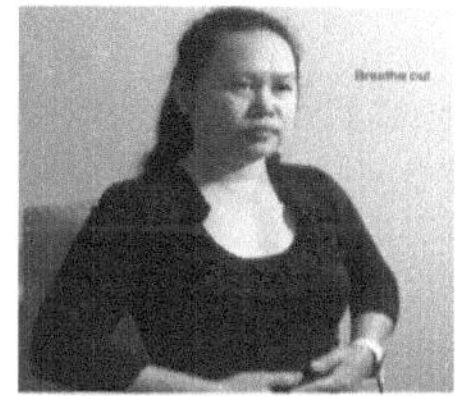

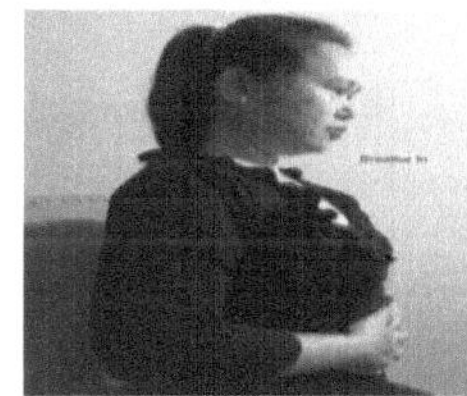

NECK EXERCISES

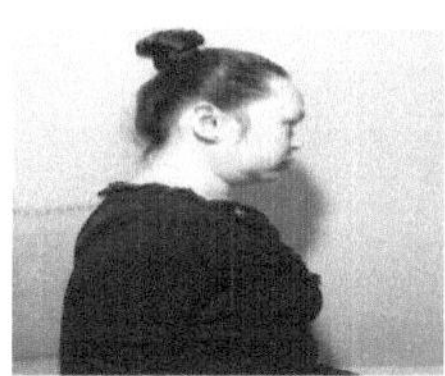

Look up & down

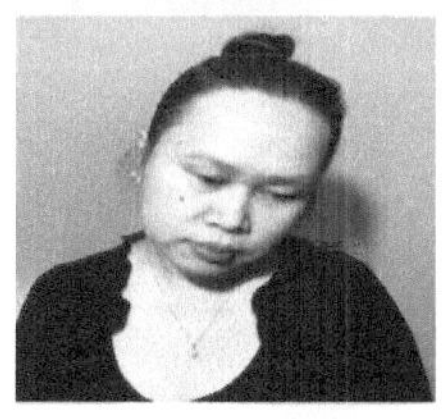

Look right/look left

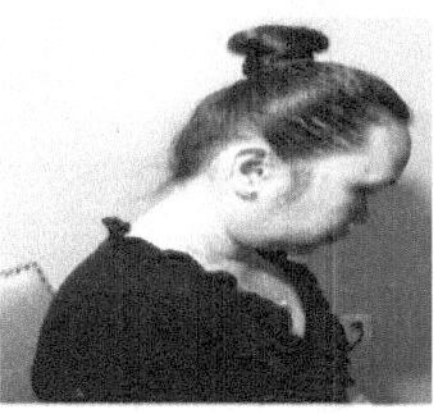

Look down

131

STICK EXERCISES

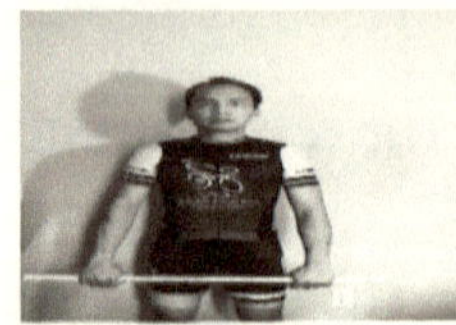

Stick down

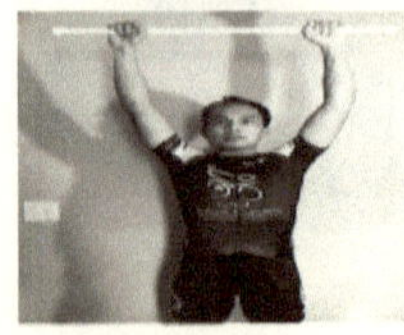

Raise stick up

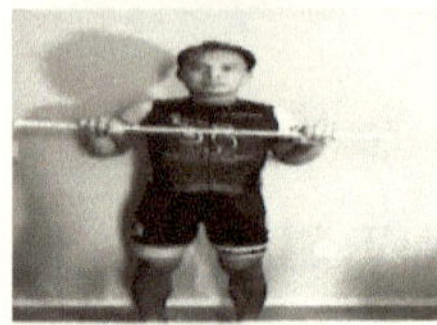

Stick from chest

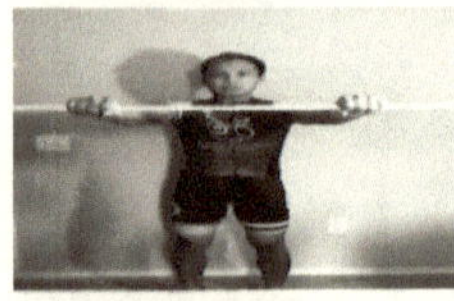

Stick away from the chest

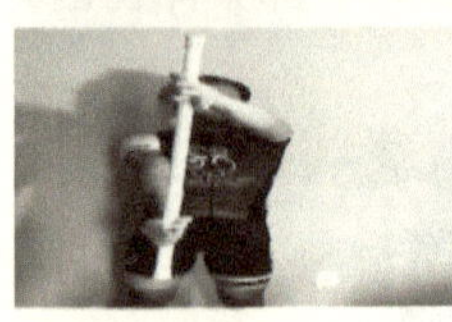

Stick canoe/row

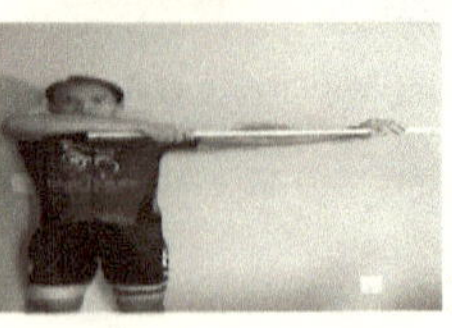

Move stick sideways

LOWER BODY EXERCISES

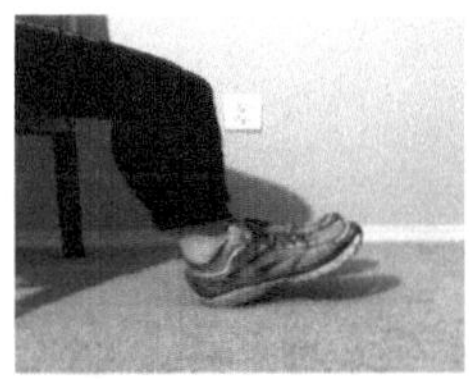

Toes up

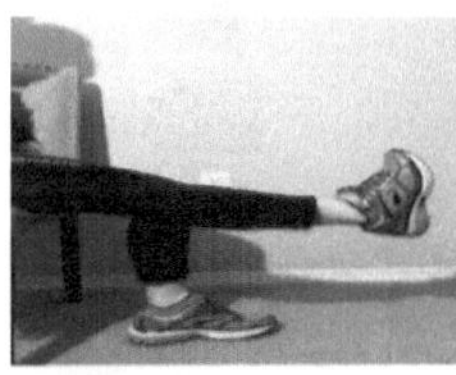

Leg kick forward

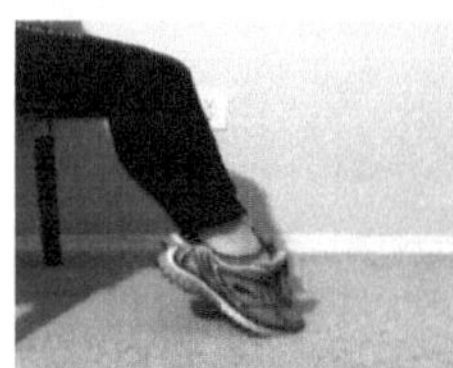

Heel raises

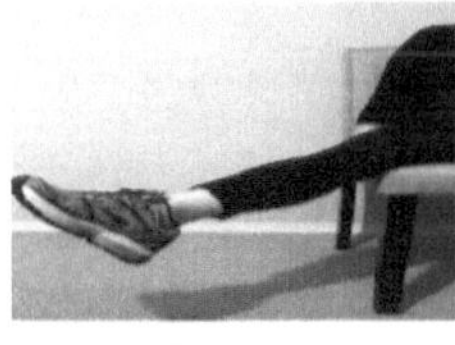

Leg kick sideways

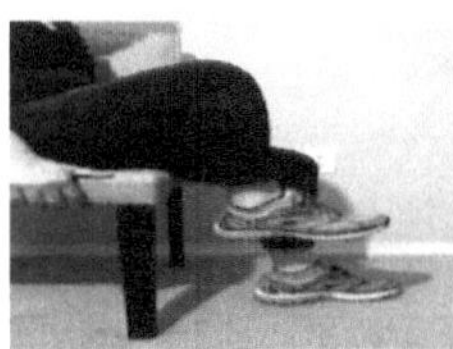

Knee raises

Upper Body Exercises

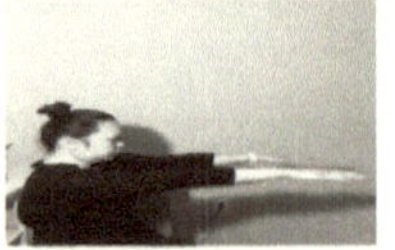

Arms forward

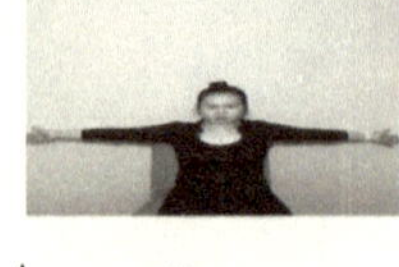

Arms out

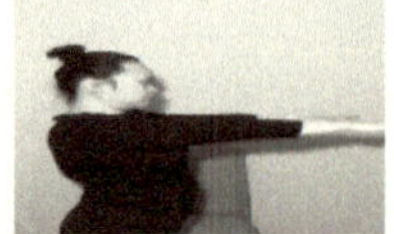

Elbows straight

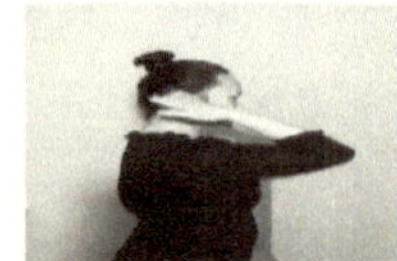

Elbows Bend

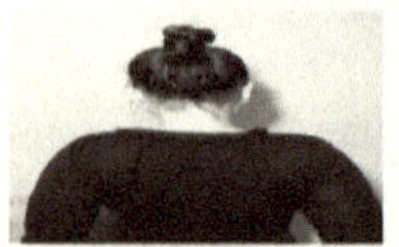

Shoulder Blade squeezes

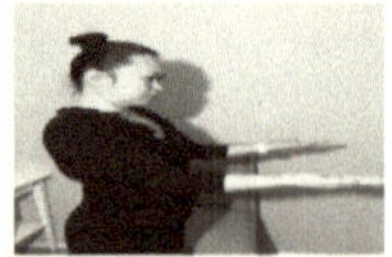

Palms up

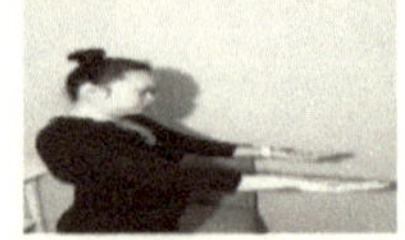

Palms down

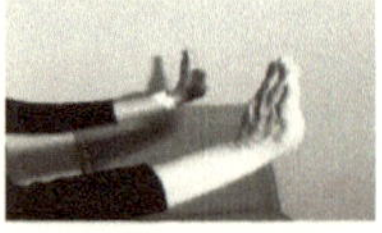

Wrists up

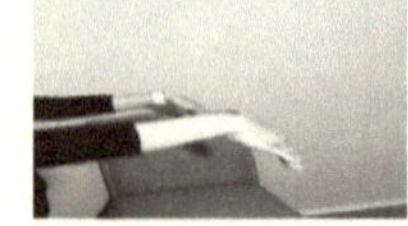

Wrists down

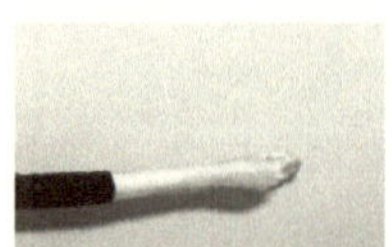

Make a fist

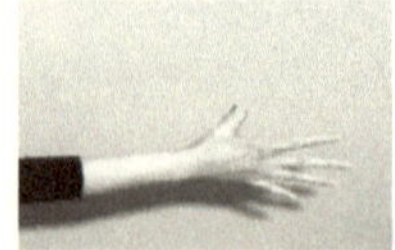

Fingers opened

OTHER TYPES OF EXERCISES

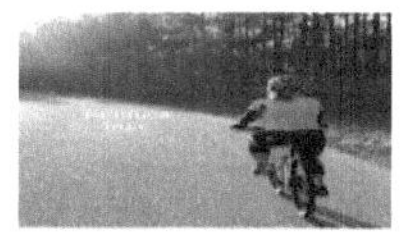

Biking

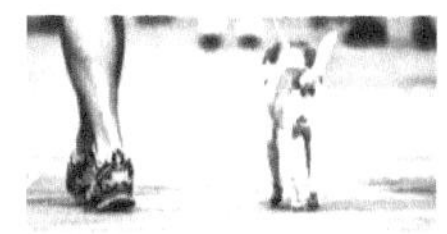

Brisk Walking

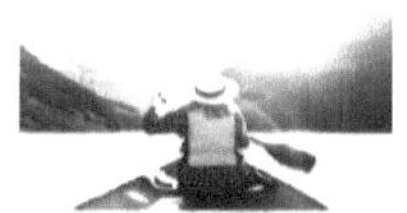

Canoing (when able)

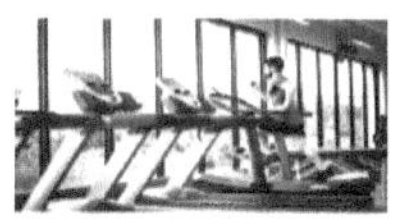

Treadmill

CHAPTER 9

ADJUCTIVE THERAPY POPULARLY USED BY SOME LYMPHEDEMA WARRIORS

KINESIOTAPING

The kinesiotaping (KT) technique has become famous for the reduction in the size of a lymphedematous limb in the early stages of breast cancer-related lymphedema. KT increases lymph flow and can be used in the treatment of peripheral lymphedema. It is applied to the skin to make a gentle push on the skin, which then causes the lymphatic vessels under the skin to absorb and drain the lymph fluid from the swollen areas into the areas with sufficient or normal lymphatic drainage.

According to the study conducted by Malicka et al., the primary goal of KT is to reroute the flow of lymph from an area of congestion or swelling towards the place of the normal lymphatic flow to obtain a decrease in the volume of the edema.

Some advantages of KT according to this study includes:

1. A relief of pain or abnormal sensation, improvement in muscle function, get rid of lymph accumulating under the skin, and improves joint integrity.

2. KT increases the space between the skin and muscle tissue, which facilitates blood and lymph flow.

3. It is better tolerated by patients and can be worn for 1-3 days or longer. It is similar to lymphatic drainage, though it allows patients to receive therapeutic benefits 24 hours a day.

4. Kinesiology Taping applications pull the skin slightly, creating more space between the dermis and fascia.

5. KT is more similar to compression therapy in that it reduces capillary filtration rather than enhancing lymphangiomotor function.

6. One disadvantage of KT is that the skin is at a higher risk of getting wounds.

7. KT might be a more useful option for patients with poor tolerance of bandaging, as it is more comfortable to the skin especially in hot climates and during the summer.

8. It is a simpler and less demanding technique than compression bandaging, which prompts the patient's compliance.

Research 1:

A randomized, cross-over, controlled trial by Pajero Otero et al. was conducted to show the efficacy of Kinesio taping compared to compression garments during the maintenance phase of complex decongestive therapy for breast cancer-related lymphedema.

The participants of the study were divided into two groups; one receiving Kinesio taping and the other with a compression garment, both wore them for four weeks. A four-week washout period was established prior to the interventions and between them.

The study has shown that Kinesio taping was more effective than compression garments in decreasing the volume of lymphedema and had less severe lymphedema-related symptoms such as pain, tightness, heaviness, and hardness; improvement of upper-limb mobility, and are more comfortable.

Research 2:

It has been observed that upper extremity lymphedema is one of the riskiest and most common complications following breast cancer surgery that increases the likelihood of functional impairment, psychological, and social problems.

Tantawy et al. performed a comparative randomized controlled trial between the effects of Kinesio taping (KT) and pressure garment (PG) on Secondary Upper Extremity Lymphedema and Quality of Life Following Mastectomy.

The purpose of this study is to compare the effects of kinesiotaping versus compression garments in Breast cancer UE secondary lymphedema. There were 66 female participants. The KT group (33) received Kinesio taping application (2 times per week for three weeks), while the PG group (33) received pressure garment (20- 60 mmHg) for at least 15-18 hours per day for three weeks.

The results of their study showed that the KT group had more improvement in limb circumference, SPADI (shoulder pain disability index), handgrip strength, and overall quality of life than the PG group at the end of the intervention.

Research 3:

Another investigative study of Ergin et al. on the effect of using Kinesio Taping (KT) on anastomotic regions along with complex decongestive physiotherapy (CDP) in patients with breast cancer-related lymphedema (BCRL). In this study two groups were compared: Group 1 (CDP only, n= 14) and Group 2(CDP + KT n=18). The outcome measure was the difference in the reduction of limb volumes between the groups.

CDP included manual lymphatic drainage, compression bandages, exercises, and skincare. KT was applied to the lymphatic anastomosis. All patients received treatment for 1 hour per day, five days per week, for four weeks. Surprisingly, the study has shown that applying KT to lymphatic anastomotic regions is not effective in reducing limb volume in the management of breast cancer related lymphedema.

DRY BRUSHING

Schwartz et al. stated that dry brushing is a massage technique used in Ayurvedic medicine that originated in India 5,000 years ago. The people in India believed that dry brushing is used to relieve lymphatic congestion that causes stress and diseases. It has also been commonly used to decrease lymphedema and inflammation from lymphatic filariasis.

Lymphatic filariasis is a parasitic disease caused by microscopic, thread-like worms that only live in the human lymph system.

141

Interestingly, the sports industry, which has been interested in promoting post-training recovery and reducing edema, is investigating the utility of peristaltic pulse dynamic compression (PPDC) devices that simulate manual lymphatic therapies. Recently, this device was shown to increase the "pressure-to-pain threshold" in elite athletes and also to induce the anti-inflammatory genes, but it is unclear whether these effects are can help improve lymphatic flow. Furthermore, there is an evident potential for the lymphatic massage technique using dry brushing could be used to improve lymphatic function to help reduce tissue inflammation in autoimmune diseases.

There are some products available in the internet for dry brush that some lymphedema warriors are using for self-brushing techniques at home. Below is a link to the amazon website that you can purchase brushes at a good price. Check at: https://amzn.to/2Ye7ALz

CHAPTER 10

COMMONLY ASKED QUESTIONS ABOUT LYMPHEDEMA

What is lymphedema?

A medical condition is an abnormal swelling of the extremities, trunk and other body parts due to the failure of the lymphatic system to eliminate lymph into the circulation. It is an abnormal build-up of protein-rich fluid in the outside of the tissue cells of the body.

What is lipedema?

Lipedema is a chronic condition that occurs most commonly in women with a symmetrical presentation of painful fat buildup and swelling in the lower body and with no affectation of the hands and feet.

What is a lymphatic system?

Your lymphatic system is crucial to keeping your body healthy. It circulates protein-rich lymph fluid throughout your body, collecting bacteria, viruses, and waste products. Your lymphatic system carries this fluid and harmful substances through your lymph vessels, which lead to lymph nodes. The wastes are then filtered out by lymphocytes — infection-fighting cells that live in your lymph nodes — and ultimately flushed from your body.

What are lymph nodes?

Lymph nodes are small sac-like structures located along lymph vessels. The lymphocytes which are types of white blood cell lives here > They control the immune responses by allowing lymphocytes to come into contact with foreign materials.

How many lymph nodes are there in a human body?

There are 500 to 600 lymph nodes distributed throughout the body, with clusters found in the armpit, groin, neck, chest and abdomen.

What are the stages of lymphedema?

Stage 0 no visible edema, has an injury to the lymphatic system

Stage 1 visible edema pitting

Stage 2 visible edema nonpitting

Stage 3 visible edema with skin discoloration and thickening

· Swelling of a part or all of your arm or leg, toes or fingers

· A feeling of heaviness or tightness

· Restricted range of motion

· Pain, aching or discomfort

· Recurring infections

· Fibrosis or hardening and thickening of the skin

Lymphedema occurs when the lymphatic system functions in an abnormal manner due to injuries from surgery or from anomalies in the system, then lymphedema occurs.

Causes of secondary lymphedema:

· Surgery. Removal of or damage to lymph nodes and lymph vessels may result in lymphedema. For example, lymph nodes may be removed to check for the spread of breast cancer, and lymph nodes may be injured in surgery that involves blood vessels in your limbs.

· Radiation treatment for cancer. Radiation can cause scarring and inflammation of your lymph nodes or lymph vessels.

· Cancer. If cancer cells block lymphatic vessels, lymphedema may result. Such as, when a tumor growing near a lymph node or lymph vessel could enlarge enough to prevent the flow of the lymph fluid.

· Infection. An infection of the lymph nodes or infection caused by parasites that can restrict the flow of lymph fluid. It is most common in developing countries in the tropical and subtropical regions.

Causes of primary lymphedema:

Primary lymphedema is a rare, inherited condition caused by problems with the development of lymph vessels in your body.

Specific causes of primary lymphedema include:

· A congenital lymphedema or Milroy's disease. An anomaly or disorder that starts in infancy and causes lymph nodes to form abnormally.

· Lymphedema praecox or Meige's disease. A type of lymphedema that occurs during puberty or during pregnancy, and may also occur later, until age 35.

· A lymphedema tarda or late-onset lymphedema. It usually begins after age 35 and is not a common form of lymphedema.

How is lymphedema diagnosed?

If you're at risk of lymphedema because you just had a surgery that involves removing your lymph nodes or cutting parts of the lymphatic system, such as for clients with cancer surgeries, then your doctor may diagnose lymphedema based on your signs and symptoms and the history of lymph node removal.

However, if the cause of your lymphedema is not from a surgical procedure, then the doctor may order some imaging tests to investigate your lymphatic system to rule out lymphedema.

Some tests to diagnose lymphedema:

147

· **MRI scan.**

· **CT scan.** It can reveal blockages in the lymphatic system.

· **Doppler ultrasound.** The conventional ultrasound looks at blood flow and pressure by using high-frequency sound waves from the ultrasound machine off red blood cells to help find obstructions and detects blood clots.

· **Lymphoscintigraphy** is a radionuclide imaging of your lymphatic system. A radioactive dye is injected in the system and then scanned by a machine. The resulting images will show the dye moving through your lymph vessels and can highlight the blockages.

· **Infections.** Cellulitis or bacterial infection of the skin and lymphangitis or infection of the lymph vessels. Even the smallest injury to your arm or leg can be an entry point for infection.

· **Lymphangiosarcoma.** A rare form of soft tissue cancer can result from the most severe cases of untreated lymphedema. Some possible signs of lymphangiosarcoma include blue-red or purple marks on the skin.

148

What are some early signs and symptoms of
lymphedema?

Lymphedema signs and symptoms, which occur in your affected arm or leg, include:

· Swelling of part or all of your arm or leg, including fingers or toes

· Heaviness or tightness of the arm or leg

· Restricted range of motion

· Aching or discomfort

· Recurring infections

· Hardening or thickening of the skin (fibrosis)

The swelling caused by lymphedema ranges from mild, hardly noticeable changes in the size of your arm or leg to extreme changes that make the limb challenging to use.

Lymphedema caused by cancer treatment may not occur until months or years after treatment.

When to see a doctor or lymphedema therapist?

Make an appointment with your doctor if you notice persistent swelling in your arm or leg, weeping or leaking of water on your arms or legs, redness of the skin, swelling of legs that does not go away with elevation.

If you already have the diagnosis of lymphedema of a limb, see your doctor if there is a sudden dramatic increase in the size of the involved limb, as it may suggest a new process is occurring.

Is this condition preventable?

Lymphedema is preventable through the gold standard of treatment, which is complete decongestive therapy.

If you have had or you are going to have cancer surgery, ask your doctor whether your procedure will involve your lymph nodes or lymph vessels. Ask if your radiation treatment will be aimed at lymph nodes, so you'll be aware of the possible risks.

What are the DO's and DON'Ts of lymphedema?

DO's:

· Protect your arm or leg.

150

· Protect yourself from sharp objects. For example, shave with an electric razor, wear gloves when you garden or cook, and use a thimble when you sew.

· Rest your arm or leg while recovering.

· After cancer treatment, exercise and stretching are encouraged.

· Avoid heat on your arm or leg. Also, protect your affected limb from extreme cold.

· Elevate your arm or leg. Whenever possible, elevate your affected limb above the level of your heart.

· Avoid tight clothing. Avoid anything that could constrict your arm or leg, such as tightfitting clothing and, in the case of your arm, blood pressure cuffs. Ask that your blood pressure be taken in your other arm.

- Keep your arm or leg clean.
- Make skin and nail care high priorities.
- Inspect the skin on your arm or leg daily, watching for changes or breaks in your skin that could lead to infection.

DON'TS:

- Don't go barefoot.

· Don't apply ice or heat, such as with a heating pad, to your affected limb.

· Avoid strenuous activity until you've recovered from surgery or radiation.

· If possible, avoid medical procedures, such as blood draws and vaccinations, in your affected limb.

· Avoid injury to your affected limb. Cuts, scrapes, and burns can invite infection.

What are the ages commonly affected by lymphedema?

Lymphedema affects children, teenagers, middle-aged, and elderly.

What is the incidence /epidemiology of lymphedema?

Tan et al. indicated in 2011 that one in every 30 individuals globally is affected by LE.

The incidence of lymphedema is fifty percent in breast cancer patients, and sixty-four percent in cancer patients that underwent radiation and surgical removal of the axillary lymph node and pelvic lymph node.

There is a low incidence rate among children and adults with "congenital or hereditary lymphovascular defects."

The secondary lymphedema approximately affects 90% in the world (Park et al., 2016).

In the research done by Ross in 2016, in the United States of America, the primary lymphedema is most often encountered by one of every 10,000 persons, and eighty percent have lymphedema praecox. Additionally, basing on the research study conducted by Boneti, Arentz, & Klimberg in 2010, lymphedema in the US is most commonly seen in postsurgical removal of lymph nodes in breast cancer, and the incidence rate is increased if they received radiation therapy postoperatively, and 10-40% will have lymphedema in the ipsilateral arm.

Moreover, females are most often affected by primary lymphedema, and 70% to 80% of congenital lymphedema (i.e., the LE praecox often occurs in 1 of every 100,000 females and 1 in 400,000 males.

Complete decongestive therapy is the gold standard of lymphedema treatment.

There are some drugs that most often recommended and prescribed by primary doctors. Diuretics are very well-known medication for edema, however; the majority does not believe that this medication is effective and can lead to worsening of symptoms of uncomplicated lymphedema. The drug will only remove the water component of the edema while the protein remains in the tissue, which continues to draw water back towards the cells when the drug's potency is gone.

Benzopyrones are also known drug for treating lymphedema in other countries. They are shown to stimulate the macrophage activity of the cells to fight infection and can separate the proteins in the lymph fluid. However, the effects are minimal and can take six months to show a decrease in size or volume. The drug is not FDA approved here in the USA, only in Australia Europe since the 1980s.

In the systematic review performed by Badger et all, they found out that due to a decrease infiltration, the drugs have some positive effects on pain and discomfort in the swollen areas; however, some cases of liver toxicity were found. Overall, between the placebo and active participants, there was no difference in findings; that is why this drug has not been approved by the FDA.

Another study by Forte et al., on the use of pharmacotherapy agents in treating lymphedema patients with anti-inflammatory drugs, have shown that some promising outcomes in using Ketoprofen, selenium, and tacrolimus. WebMD stated that ***Ketoprofen*** is approved by the US FDA for chronic forms of inflammation like arthritis, however, in using it for lymphedema appears to alleviate the burden of the condition in a small study conducted by Stanford University researchers.

What are the surgical options for lymphedema?

The ***Charles procedure*** is the oldest and the most radical ablative procedure. It was generally done for patients with advanced-stage lymphedema, debilitating lymphedema that does not respond to complete decongestive therapy, and elephantiasis. The main goal is to control and eradicate infection while simultaneously reducing excessive volume.

The ***modified Charles' procedure***, on the other hand, entails the preservation of the greater saphenous vein and its superficial branches. The greater saphenous vein and its branches can be used later as a recipient drain for a transferred lymph node. Patients with severe lower extremity lymphedema may benefit from the combination of vascularized lymph node and modified Charles' procedure.

Radical Reduction in Lymphedema with Preservation of Perforators

This procedure combines both approaches, excisional and microsurgical principles to manage lymphedema. The advantage of this procedure is that it allows for more aggressive debulking of the lymphedematous tissue without damaging essential perforators. The disadvantages, however, lie in the fact that such procedure leaves unsightly scars, prolonged operating time, risk of infection, skin breakdown, and necrosis.

SAL (Suction Assisted Lipectomy)

It is the least invasive procedure for lymphedema. It has the most minimal morbidity and highest patient satisfaction when compared with other ablative procedures. The only disadvantage of this procedure is that patients must wear compression garments immediately following the procedure.

Excisional procedures have been described for the management of lymphedema since early 1900. Despite the advancements made and the advent of microsurgical techniques, these procedures remain relevant and can be performed to reduce morbidity, risk of infection, and improve quality of life. It can be done when the physiologic methods do not offer adequate relief or satisfactory results.

Vascularized Lymph Node Transfer

VLNT is an alternative physiologic procedure that can improve lymph drainage flow, in patients where, functional lymphatic channels are absent or dysfunctional, such as

157

following lymphadenectomy or radiotherapy. The exact mechanism is still unknown, and several theories have been proposed. Most likely, the mechanism of action is a combination of those theories. The first theory is that the lymph node absorbs the excess lymphatic fluid accumulating in the vicinity. The second theory is the vascularized lymph nodes generates lymphangiogenesis by releasing vascular endothelial growth factor-C.

Lymphovenous Anastomosis

LVA is a procedure where the excess lymph is directed into the venous circulation. The surgeon will connect a lymph vessel in the affected leg or arm or affected area to a nearby vein to bypass the damaged area and restores the flow of lymph fluid to the venous system.

Is there a diet to follow to fight for this lymphedema?

There is no specific diet for lymphedema. But experts and researches showed that maintaining a healthy body mass index and average body weight is essential to prevent an increase in the severity of lymphedema and to keep the smallest size and volume of edema that can be self-managed

158

to avoid risks of infections and other complications. Please refer to the Diet and Nutrition Chapter of this book for some recommendations.

One can be a certified lymphedema therapist through a comprehensive training seminar which is a combination of hands-on training and lectures and one has to undergo a certification examination to be fully certified. Some of the famous schools you can enroll and get your certification are the following:

Academy of Lymphatic Studies (ACOLS).

Norton School of Lymphatic Therapy.

Klose Training Lymphedema Certification.

International Lymphedema and Wound Training Institute.

You can search in your local area for a certified lymphedema therapist. The majority of the vascular surgeon,

159

wound care doctors, cardiologists, and primary doctors are very aware of this condition. They can help you find a therapist that can perform lymphedema therapy for you. You can also search the web, below is the website you can browse, or you can type in the google web search "Find lymphedema therapist in my area." or use the tool below.

https://www.acols.com/find-therapist/
https://lymphaticnetwork.org/living-with-lymphedema/find-a-lymphedema-therapist/

I am bigger than my lymphedema.

I am not my struggle.

I will survive this and will overcome it.

I will keep moving forward.

Nothing will keep me down.

I will rebuild myself stronger than before.

Anonymous

CHAPTER 11

BECOMING A LYMPHEDEMA WARRIOR

"He who conquers himself is the mightiest warrior."
Confucius

The best narrators and authors are the survivors or the people living with the medical condition. They are the ones that can explain to someone everything about the disease or issues that they have through their experiences and their fight to continue to live a life with quality despite the constant effects of the problem—a quality of life in their unique way.

A few of the stories of lymphedema warriors I have met.

Disclaimer: All narration is for story purposes only. No names or locations were written for privacy. The stories are not specifics but are general circumstances and encounters the author experienced.

Warrior #1

"To accept reality is the first step of winning the battle."I.E.

A charming young-elderly retired teacher one day came to my care. She was a breast cancer survivor who had a mastectomy and was advised to seek consultation for her upper extremity lymphedema. Her story struck home for me. She has always been living a healthy lifestyle, exercising, eating healthy, and enjoying life with her spouse. Then one day, the news which nobody on earth wants to hear came. Her doctor said, "you have breast cancer stage 2." It was like a series of lightning that hit her in the chair she was sitting in the doctor's office, with her husband sitting on her side. It was news and hoping it was a fake one. Some of the hardest reality in life is facing a situation that is dreaded. It is the exact opposite feeling of winning the lottery or hearing your first child's cry and seeing his or her beautiful face. But life has to go on! She has to move on and has to continue to hear the sad reality. Her doctor explained her plan of care, of how she is going to fight and kick this disease out of her way, and now, it is! She has always been a fighter. She had the mastectomy done and was referred to a lymphedema therapist while she had been undergoing radiation therapy treatment. It took her a while to get started with lymphedema therapy for both arms as the surgeon can't find a therapist near her until finally, they were able to reach me, and she became my client. Before seeing her, she was already researching information about lymphedema of her arms related to her mastectomy. She is like a girl scout, always prepared, and will do the best to find the best therapy she can have. She is a warrior fighting this new condition and with her breast cancer.

Warrior #2

"Consistency and determination to win are some of the greatest qualities of a soldier."

Another lady came to the clinic one day. She was limping on her right leg while walking at the entrance of the clinic. She is a tall lady who has a slender body stature, a young-looking elderly in her late 70's. She was sent by her primary doctor to assess her right leg swelling that never goes down no matter how much she elevates her leg at night or sitting in a recliner chair. She has no history of circulation issues nor recent surgery. Upon questioning and talking to the lady, she mentioned that she had a vein stripping procedure on the

164

back of her right thigh that was causing pain and discomfort. Has prompted her to seek medical advice through the vascular surgeon. A few months after surgery, the doctor referred her to the lymphedema therapist for further evaluation of her leg swelling that lingered, although the pain has subsided on her thigh. The client narrated that her mom and grandma had the same problem when they were in their late 60's. Diagnostic tests and imaging performed, and she was found out to have primary lymphedema of the right side of her leg. So, lymphedema therapy was started, proper education and training were given, and the patient was able to digest the reasons for her leg edema. She went back to playing golf as her passion and was not scared of doing so as long as she does her home therapy and wears stockings like a true lymph warrior. It never stopped her from doing things that she loves to do. And her life continued, knowing the right medical condition and the right therapy is a big help to her journey. She will be a warrior of keeping daily care of her lymphie leg.

Warrior #3

"A lot of warriors are made by their life's struggles."

165

All of us are warriors. Not only this affects the female population, but also the masculine gender is not spared. Mr. M. was under my care at home for physical therapy due to difficulty in walking. Upon evaluation, he was found out to have a longtime history of both lower legs swelling and thickened and hardened skin of both lower limbs. He said that when he was in his late 50's, he had a surgical procedure to remove the cancerous tumor cells on his pelvic region, and the doctor has to remove ten inguinal lymph nodes on both sides. He had undergone radiation therapy on both inguinal and pelvic areas. The swelling slowly build-up as the years went by, until after ten years later his leg is getting so big and bulky that it is so difficult for him to walk and he had several bouts of leg redness and infection prompting several hospital admissions. He was given proper education and training on the disease and its prognosis and the outcome of his leg swelling. The complete decongestive therapy was performed on both phases, and now he and his spouse are well trained in self-management. He continues to be a warrior of his lymphedema, and the fight is not over it.

Warrior #4

"I don't have a disability, but I have an inability to refuse to enjoy my ability."I.E

An elderly lady in her late 70's I have known in the past during one of my home health therapy. She was referred for physical therapy due to a recent decline in her functional mobility with a longtime history of stroke and a left-sided weakness. Upon assessment, she also has right lower extremity lymphedema due to right inguinal lymph node biopsy and removal of cancerous nodes, which caused her right leg lymphedema. The lady loves to walk with her wide-based quad cane despite her weakness she manages to enjoy her daily walk outside her house. When one walks with one side of her body is functioning only fifty percent, we know how determined they are. And she is this person.

A born warrior will fight to stay healthy and enjoy their life to give quality to it, no matter what status it is at the moment. She was very diligent in doing her self-lymphedema management. She does her compression pump daily at least 2 hours a day, and always wore her compression stockings to keep the leg in an average volume. Despite her left-sided weakness from her stroke, she never gives up in taking care of her right leg lymphedema.

Warrior #5

"When I accepted that it is okay not to be okay, then I became stronger."I.E.

A retired medical technologist once was under my care for lipedema and lymphedema of both lower extremities and abdomen. She lives alone in a single-story house with short-term caregiver assistance three to four times a week to help with house chores and assist in her daily living activities. She was hesitant to believe that she can continue to live with her condition. Depression and anxiety soaked her body and soul. Life has its little miracles and she did have her dose of it. She woke up one day and told herself, I need to do something so win over this disease. I am stronger than this and I am always a positive strong person. I will fight no matter what it takes.

She religiously follows all treatment regimen to keep her edema and swelling at a size that will keep her going with

168

her everyday life. Her abdominal edema and morbid obesity were limiting her quality of life and mobility inside her house. She never gave up. She walks even if it hurts. And she refused to use a wheelchair and live her life to the fullest while consistently doing her complete decongestive therapy. She was a warrior and never a sign of giving up in her system.

Warrior # 6

"The heart of a child is a warrior in disguise. "I.E.

Another warrior is a delightful young, older adult who had a traumatic brain injury when he was in his first decade of life. Since he was born, he has been experiencing God's miracles that kept him going with his life. He is the youngest child in his family. The one accident that changed his life made him and his family more robust than ever. I met Mr. J a few years ago for physical therapy in his lovely home near the Florida waters. He had a right-sided weakness as a residual deficit of his accident as a child. I never thought that I would see him again and, at this time, as one of my lymphedema warriors. His family reported that his legs had

169

been swollen on and off for a couple of years now. And they have seen by a vascular doctor once and was referred to a lymphedema clinic. He was only seen earlier in the clinic, and then his family has been doing his leg bandaging. Our paths led again to each other when he was referred by his orthopedic surgeon for physical therapy and lymphedema therapy. He is one of my best clients that never questions about his therapy. He enjoys all his treatment and happy always to see results that range from a small win to a huge success. He is born a warrior from all of his medical issues and his big heart. He is not a quitter. He is always up and going and is willing to follow therapy protocols to keep his quality of life and enjoy it.

Warrior # 7

"I am mightier than my cancer."

A charming older woman who came into my care for a status post radiation treatment for her right breast cancer was another cancer and lymphedema warrior. She also had SP right mastectomy, obesity, and a history of chronic back and leg pain. She was referred under my care for home health services for her right UE and left UE lymphedema SP right breast mastectomy and axillary node removal. The patient has been having pain issues with her back, hips, knee, and lower leg. She takes care of her spouse, who has early-onset dementia. She has gone into depression with her new diagnosis but is willing to fight to the end to learn how to live with her lymphedema, cancer, and chronic pain. She said, "nothing can stop me from living my life and taking care of my family." She had great success with her therapy and was discharged from my care.

Warrior # 8

"I am a patient, I am a caregiver, and I am excited to take care of my legs, so I can continue to enjoy my everyday activities."

Another very pleasant elderly lady with bilateral foot and lower leg edema was referred for evaluation and assessment of her leg swelling and decline in all her functional status. She lives with her spouse, who has multiple chronic issues, which makes her the primary caregiver. They have a house caretaker as needed, but she does most of the community's access despite her condition. She tolerated the complete decongestive therapy well and was very happy for the results of her leg size going down and getting lighter. She managed to learn how to do her self-bandaging, wear her compression garments at night, and use her compression pump daily as instructed. The patient has a full understanding that her self-management has to be a part of her daily routine to avoid complications and recurring problems of swelling and infection. "I will do whatever I can to the best of my ability while I can do this, I will do my part." A quote from this elderly lymphedema warrior.

Warrior #9

"I will stand up every time I fall. There is no stopping me from enjoying my noontime TV show."

A retired nurse who has been living with both lower leg lymphedema told her story of what it feels like to be in her shoe to have lymphedema. She has histories of low blood pressure, low oxygen saturation upon ambulation and standing, and bad vertigo and dizzy spells. She remains active at home, whether in her wheelchair or walking very short distances using her two-wheeled walker for safety.

Living alone with her cats and dogs, she describes her leg edema as a significant hindrance in her ability to do more at home, which made her paralyzed in doing household chores with no issues. And with her vertigo and dizziness, all functional mobility and activities of daily living are so challenging to perform. However, this patient does not mind wearing her leg compression bandages and using her leg pump to keep her swelling down, not blowing up, and get skin infection or cellulitis. She narrated that her leg started giving her issues with swelling and heaviness five years ago. It started giving her problems when she was hospitalized for her dizziness and was admitted to the skilled nursing facility. The admission made her less mobile and made her leg bigger and heavier. Later, one of her doctors told her she has lymphedema and needs to be evaluated by a certified therapist for the problem. Then commences her journey of lymphedema therapy. Until she was discharged home, received continued treatment, and was taught and trained by her therapist in self-management of her condition as it is going to be a long-term issue is not curable but preventable.

Warrior # 10

173

"I am bigger than my pain, and this is not going to stop me from going."

I still remember my very first client for both lower leg lymphedema, a very pleasant morbidly obese lady due to thyroid issues, and multiple medical comorbidities. She lived in the countryside of town with her significant other in a mobile home with five steps in the entrance of the house with handrails. The patient was very cooperative and compliant with her lymphedema therapy. She never missed a scheduled visit even if she is not feeling well at times. She wanted to make sure she will get compression bandages as prescribed for her to improve her quality of life and perform her daily activities with no problem. And most notably, she always says, I would like to keep my leg edema down as much as possible to avoid risks of me going to the hospital. The patient has chronic pain on all her joints and wearing her leg bandages was a significant burden to her mobility. However, she will not mind the pain and the heaviness because she knows that this treatment is for her to keep her lymphedema at a normal volume or size to prevent complications of infection, falls, and injuries, and to avoid any feared hospital stays. She is a lymphedema warrior fighting and living the condition with grace and dignity.

" The true warrior understands and seizes that moment by giving an effort so intense and so intuitive that it could only be called one from the heart".

Pat Riley

175

CHAPTER 12
SAMPLE HEALTH AND WELLNESS FOR LYMPHEDEMA

Prevention is the best medication. A concept that has been proven to be effective in decreasing mortality and improving once quality of life. Health promotion to prevent injuries and diseases that can be debilitating are one of the issues solved by health and wellness promotion. Edintong et.al, stated in their journal about health promotion for the 21st century that all health care providers including can help patients find the right resources to support their health and well-being in the workplace, in their communities, and within their own families. And most importantly, the provision of highest quality of support and care for the health and well-being of patients will require better understanding of the many possible social and environmental determinants of sickness, health, and flourishing. Below is a sample Health & Wellness promotion program for lymphedema.

I. DIET/NUTRITION

1. Good proper hydration
2. Good nutrition/proper diet plans

3. Taking prescribed medications and over-the-counter supplements. Do not self-medicate.

II.   DAILY EXERCISES

1. Walking outdoor and indoor treadmill (30 minutes)

2. Road biking, fitness bike or stationary bike rides (30 minutes)

3. Range of motion exercises using cane or stick, Thera-band exercises

4. Weights and strengthening exercises

5. Pilates, Yoga, Tai Chi exercises

III.   DAILY SELF MLD

Start from neck, to upper body, trunk and lower body MLD exercises daily.

IV: DAILY LEG PUMP

Use your upper body, trunk or leg pumps daily 1 to 2 hours as tolerated.

V: DAILY SKIN CARE

Daily skin care either taking a shower, daily leg or arm washing using low Ph soap or soap substitutes, and make sure to dry skin thoroughly and use low Ph lotion.

177

VI: CONTINUING TO EDUCATE SELF ON LYMPHEDEMA

Read books, magazines, articles, and blogs and watch reliable videos about lymphedema and get help from your local lymphedema therapists and doctors to further assess your condition.

VIII: JOIN SUPPORT GROUP (KNOW YOURE NOT ALONE)

Some great groups to join: Lymphedema Stand Up Strong FB group. Lymphedema support group. LEARN group. Go on Facebook and Instagram and find your tribe. It really helps a lot in learning and knowing that you are not alone in your journey and in living a life as a lymphedema warrior.

IX: CALLING YOUR THERAPIST/PRIMARY CARE PHYSICIAN FOR ANY CHANGE IN MEDICAL STATUS AND LYMPHEDEMA STATUS.

Prevention is the best cure. Call for help through your therapists and doctors if you are not sure what is going on to be evaluated properly and to receive proper care sooner

RECORDS OF MY MEDICAL HISTORIES, S/S, COMPLAINTS

SIGNS/SYMPTOM S	ONSET

HEALTH & WELLNESS CHART FOR LYMPHEDEMA

	HEALTH & WELLNESS PROGRAM
MY LYMPHEDEMA	AGE: WT: HT:
	Edema Size:
	Affected area
DIET & NUTRITION	Hydration:
	Diet:
	Breakfast:
	Lunch:
	Dinner:
EXERCISES	
	Choice of exercise:
	Frequency:
SKIN CARE	Daily Washing with low ph soap
	Daily use of low ph lotion or Vaseline
SELF MANUAL LYMPHATIC DRAINAGE	Daily Self MLD exercises
COMPRESSION PUMP	Daily use of compression pump 1 to 2 hours as tolerated
EDUCATION	Daily education by reading articles, blogs, and health magazines that are reliable.

	Talk to your healthcare provider and CLTs prior to trying or experimenting on new ideas or techniques for your lymphedema
SUPPORT GROUP	Join support groups online via FB or Instagram. "Lymphedema Stand up Strong FB group"
	Join your local community support groups if there are any available in your location
LYMPHEDEMA THERAPIST/DOCTOR	Keep working with your CLT. If you don't have one, find one in your area to start working with your health and wellness care.
DME COMPANY	

MY LYMPHEDEMA HEALTH & WELLNESS JOURNEY JOURNAL

	MONDAY
DAILY MOTIVATIONAL WARRIOR'S QUOTE	"A Journey of a thousand miles begins with a single step." Lao Tzu.
SELF MLD	
SKIN CARE	
BANDAGING/STOCKINGS/GARMENTS	
COMPRESSION PUMP	
DIET & NUTRITION	
MY LYMPHIE EXERCISE	
MY PROGRESS	
MY SUPPORT GROUPS	
MY DOCTOR & LYMPHEDEMA THERAPIST	

	TUESDAY
DAILY MOTIVATIONAL WARRIOR'S QUOTE	"A warrior never worries about his fear." Carlos Castaneda.
SELF MLD	
SKIN CARE	
BANDAGING/STOCKINGS/GARMENTS	
COMPRESSION PUMP	
DIET & NUTRITION	
MY LYMPHIE EXERCISE	
MY PROGRESS	
MY SUPPORT GROUPS	
MY DOCTOR & LYMPHEDEMA THERAPIST	

WEDNESDAY

DAILY MOTIVATIONAL WARRIOR'S QUOTE	""I fight for my health every day in ways most people will not understand." Anonymous
SELF MLD	
SKIN CARE	
BANDAGING/STOCKINGS/GARMENTS	
COMPRESSION PUMP	
DIET & NUTRITION	
MY LYMPHIE EXERCISE	
MY PROGRESS	
MY SUPPORT GROUPS	
MY DOCTOR & LYMPHEDEMA THERAPIST	

	THURSDAY
DAILY MOTIVATIONAL WARRIOR'S QUOTE	"Hey warriors keep going." Anonymous."
SELF MLD	
SKIN CARE	
BANDAGING/STOCKINGS/GARMENTS	
COMPRESSION PUMP	
DIET & NUTRITION	
MY LYMPHIE EXERCISE	
MY PROGRESS	
MY SUPPORT GROUPS	
MY DOCTOR & LYMPHEDEMA THERAPIST	

<table>
<tr><td></td><td>FRIDAY</td></tr>
<tr><td>MY DAILY MOTIVATIONAL WARRIOR'S QUOTE</td><td>"How little can be done under the spirit of fear."

Florence Nightingale</td></tr>
<tr><td>SELF MLD</td><td></td></tr>
<tr><td></td><td></td></tr>
<tr><td>SKIN CARE</td><td></td></tr>
<tr><td></td><td></td></tr>
<tr><td>BANDAGING/STOCKINGS/GARMENTS</td><td></td></tr>
<tr><td></td><td></td></tr>
<tr><td>COMPRESSION PUMP</td><td></td></tr>
<tr><td></td><td></td></tr>
<tr><td>DIET & NUTRITION</td><td></td></tr>
<tr><td>MY LYMPHIE EXERCISE</td><td></td></tr>
<tr><td>MY PROGRESS</td><td></td></tr>
<tr><td>MY SUPPORT GROUPS</td><td></td></tr>
<tr><td>MY DOCTOR & LYMPHEDEMA THERAPIST</td><td></td></tr>
</table>

	SATURDAY
MY DAILY MOTIVATIONAL WARRIOR'S QUOTE	"Early to bed and early to rise makes a man healthy, wealthy, & wise." Benjamin Franklin
SELF MLD	
SKIN CARE	
BANDAGING/STOCKINGS/GARMENTS	
COMPRESSION PUMP	
DIET & NUTRITION	
MY LYMPHIE EXERCISE	
MY PROGRESS	
MY SUPPORT GROUPS	
MY DOCTOR & LYMPHEDEMA THERAPIST	

	SUNDAY
MY DAILY MOTIVATIONAL WARRIOR'S QUOTE	"Be a warrior not a worrier." Anonymous
SELF MLD	
SKIN CARE	
BANDAGING/STOCKINGS/GARMENTS	
COMPRESSION PUMP	
DIET & NUTRITION	
MY LYMPHIE EXERCISE	
MY PROGRESS	
MY SUPPORT GROUPS	
MY DOCTOR & LYMPHEDEMA THERAPIST	

WHAT I DO AND WHAT I CAN OFFER.

I offer free total body diagnostics for your physical therapy, health and wellness needs, and lymphedema therapy in the comfort of your home, through phone call or via telehealth/virtual therapy session.

We also offer telehealth virtual physical therapy visits for all lymphedema patients, physical therapy, and wellness clients. We will heal and get your condition better, so you can function normally and get back up and going with the life you love.

Here is a freebie I would like to give you for purchasing my book. You will have a free two sessions for your lymphedema evaluation and formulation of the plan of care and one free treatment session through telehealth or the phone assessment, to better fit you in your needs.

Kindly email your interest for free consultations to dr_ivyenting@smartcaringphysiodoc.com, ivyentingpt@gmail.com, and let's get started in your journey for health and wellness. Or call me at my phone number 813-4104696 to get assessed and be fitted with the program for you.

189

KINDLY LEAVE ME YOUR HONEST REVIEW

It means the world to me that you purchased and read my book! I sincerely hope that you gained something from my book that you can take away and make your life better and the lives of your friends and family better!

If you have enjoyed this book and have learned from it, it would mean everything if you would leave me a positive review. Also, I would love to get your input on anything that you really enjoyed, anything that could have been better explained, or anything you would like to see in a future book.

Kindly email your interest for free consultations to ivyentingpt@gmail.com, and let's get started in your journey of health and wellness as a lymphedema warrior.

You can visit me at my blogpost website at Smart & Caring Physio Doc Pay It forward and like my page in FB, link below.

https://www.facebook.com/Smart-Caring-Physio-Doc-Pay-It-Forward-100544488220221/?modal=admin_todo_tour

Join my FB Group "Lymphedema Stand-Up Strong" with the link below.

https://www.facebook.com/groups/987268431656247/

Sincerely,

Dr. Ivy Sardoncillo Enting

Physical therapist, Certified Lymphedema Therapist, LSVT BIG certified PT, Vestibular therapist

Co-owner of Rivyve Therapy Services LLC

IMPORTANT SUGGESTED LINKS FOR YOUR LYMPHEDEMA PRODUCTS

COMPRESSION STOCKINGS

https://amzn.to/2AdLCjK

https://amzn.to/3dLHpm5

https://amzn.to/2APO93O

https://lymphedemastore.com/compression-garments/

SOCK-AID/STOCKING-AID

https://amzn.to/2MTjcP3

https://amzn.to/3haXV0T

LOTIONS/CREAMS

https://amzn.to/3cLpr1R

https://amzn.to/3dKrIvf

https://amzn.to/2UkGv8k

https://lymphedemastore.com/skin-care-a-z/

COMPRESSION PUMP

https://amzn.to/2zeCrPC

https://amzn.to/3cL87dc

COMPRESSSION VELCRO WRAPS

https://amzn.to/2MIm6WI

https://amzn.to/2BEUeQO

https://amzn.to/2MIsOvO

https://lymphedemastore.com/search.php?search_query=juzo

COMPRESSION BANDAGES KIT

https://amzn.to/30sTs41

https://amzn.to/2YhtwFA

https://lymphedemastore.com/prepackaged-bandage-kits/

DIET AND NUTRITION

https://amzn.to/3dKEU3x

https://amzn.to/2AR0JQl

https://amzn.to/2MHQsIY

EXERCISES BOOK/TOOLS

https://amzn.to/2MH00DU

https://amzn.to/2A8Gqhk

REFERENCES

1.   About adult BMI. (2020, April 11). Centers for Disease Control and
Prevention. https://www.cdc.gov/healthyweight/assessing/bmi/adult_bmi/index.html

2.   About Lipedema — Lipedema Foundation (n.d.) Lipedema Foundation.
https://www.lipedema.org/about lipedema/?gclod=Cj0KCQjwzN71BRCOARIsAF8pjfgjfaBYxBBNZLNhW1e_q2zcFTtGOP497D5Fnx5ec4GwPro8djuEoDAaAhVyEALw_wcB

3.   Aldrich, M. B., Gross, D., Morrow, J. R., Fife, C. E., & Rasmussen, J. C. (2017). Effect of pneumatic compression therapy on lymph movement in lymphedema-affected extremities, as assessed by near-infrared fluorescence lymphatic imaging. Journal of Innovative Optical Health Sciences, 10(02), 1650049. https://doi.org/10.1142/s1793545816500498

4.   Badger C, et al. (n.d.). Benzo-pyrones for reducing and controlling lymphoedema of the limbs. - PubMed - NCBI. Retrieved from
https://www.ncbi.nlm.nih.gov/pubmed/15106192

5.   Boneti, C., Arentz, S., & Klimberg, V. (2010). Axillary reverse mapping (ARM) a new technique to identify and preserve lymphatics draining the arm to prevent lymphedema. Journal of Surgical Research, 158(2), 377. https://doi.org/10.1016/j.jss.2009.11.569

6.   Borman, P. (2018). Lymphedema diagnosis, treatment, and follow-up from the view point of physical medicine and rehabilitation specialists. Turkish Journal of Physical Medicine and Rehabilitation, 64(3), 179-197. https://doi.org/10.5606/tftrd.2018.3539

7.   Common Drug Shows Promise Against Lymphedema. (2018, October 18). Retrieved from https://www.webmd.com/breast-cancer/news/20181018/common-drug-shows-promise-against-lymphedema#1

8.   Ciudad P, Sabbagh MD, Agko M, et al. Surgical Management of Lower Extremity Lymphedema: A Comprehensive Review. Indian J Plast Surg. 2019;52(1):81–92. doi:10.1055/s-0039-1688537

9.   Diet review: Paleo diet for weight loss. (2019, October 28). The Nutrition

Source. https://www.hsph.harvard.edu/nutritionsource/healthy-weight/diet-reviews/paleo-diet/

10. Douglass, J., Graves, P., & Gordon, S. (2016). Self-care for management of secondary lymphedema: A systematic review. PLOS Neglected Tropical Diseases, 10(6),e0004740. https://doi.org/10.1371/journal.pntd.0004740

11. Edington, D. W., Schultz, A. B., Pitts, J. S., & Camilleri, A. (2015). The Future of Health Promotion in the 21st Century: A Focus on the Working Population. American journal of lifestyle medicine, 10(4), 242–252. https://doi.org/10.1177/1559827615605789

12.

13. Fair, S. E. (2010). Wellness and physical therapy. Jones & Bartlett Publishers.

14. Effect of pneumatic compression

15. therapy on lymph movement in lymphedema-affected extremities, as assessed by near-infrared fluorescence lymphatic imaging. (n.d.). PubMed Central (PMC). https://www.ncbi.nlm.nih.gov/pmc/articles/PMC5665410/

16. Forte, A. J., Boczar, D., Huayllani, M. T.,

17. Lu, X., & McLaughlin, S. A. (2019).
Pharmacotherapy agents in lymphedema treatment: A systematic
review. Cureus. https://doi.org/10.7759/cureus.6300

18. Ergin, G., Şahinoğlu, E., Karadibak, D., &
Yavuzşen, T. (2019). Effectiveness of Kinesio taping on
anastomotic regions in patients with breast cancer-related
lymphedema: A randomized controlled pilot
study. Lymphatic Research and Biology, 17(6), 655-
660. https://doi.org/10.1089/lrb.2019.0003

19. ResearchGate. https://www.researchgate.net/figure/
Compression-bandage-with-underpadding-and-two-
shortstretch-bandages-applied-according-to_fig3_310790018

20. Gupta, L., Khandelwal, D., Lal, P. R., Kalra, S., &
Dutta, D. (2019). Palaeolithic Diet in Diabesity and
Endocrinopathies - A Vegan's Perspective. European
endocrinology, 15(2), 77–82. doi:10.17925/EE.2019.15.2.77

21. https://www.mayoclinic.org/diseases-
conditions/lymphedema/symptoms-causes/syc-20374682

22. https://www.sciencedirect.com/topics/medicine-and-dentistry/lymphedema

23. https://www.ncbi.nlm.nih.gov/pmc/articles/PMC3595870/pdf/avd-05-139.pdf

24. (PDF) Lymphedema and nutrition: A review. (2019,

May 13). Retrieved from
https://www.researchgate.net/publication/333070045_Lymphedema_and_nutrition_A_review

25. PDF) Lymphedema and nutrition: A review. (2019, May 13). Retrieved from
https://www/researchgate.net/publication/333070045 Lymphedema and nutrition A review

26. Lymphovenous Anastomosis (surgical procedure) - MQ Health. (n.d.). Retrieved from
https://www.mqhealth.org.au/hospital-clinics/lymphoedema-clinic/procedures/lymphovenous-anastomosis-lva

27. https://www.ncbi.nlm.nih.gov/pmc/articles/PMC3595870/pdf/avd-05-139.pdf

28. Majewski-Schrage, T., & Snyder, K. (2016). The Effectiveness of Manual Lymphatic Drainage in

Patients with Orthopedic Injuries. Journal of Sport Rehabilitation, 25(1), 91-97. doi:10.1123/jsr.2014-0222

29. Masood W, Uppaluri KR. Ketogenic Diet. [Updated 2019 Mar 21]. In: StatPearls [Internet]. Treasure Island (FL): StatPearls Publishing; 2019 Jan-. Available from: https://www.ncbi.nlm.nih.gov/books/NBK499830/

30. Malicka, I., Rosseger, A., Hanuszkiewicz, J., & Woźniewski, M. (2014). Kinesiology Taping reduces lymphedema of the upper extremity in women after breast cancer treatment: a pilot study. Przeglad menopauzalny = Menopause review, 13(4), 221–226. https://doi.org/10.5114/pm.2014.44997

31. Mastectomy: A Randomized Controlled Trial. Integr Cancer Ther. 2019;18:1534735419847276. doi:10.1177/1534735419847276
28. Nutrition and weight status | Healthy people2020. (n.d.). Healthy People 2020|. https://www.healthypeople.gov/2020/topics-objectives/topic/nutrition-and-weight-status

32. Mehrara, B. J., & Greene, A. K. (2014). Lymphedema and obesity: is there a link. Plastic and reconstructive surgery, 134(1), 154e–160e. https://doi.org/10.1097/PRS.0000000000000268

33. Melam, G. R., Buragadda, S., Alhusaini, A. A., &
Arora, N. (2016). Effect of complete decongestive
therapy and home program on health-
related quality of life in post mastectomy
lymphedema patients. BMC Women's Health, 16(1).
https://doi.org/10.1186/s12905-016-0303-9

34. Oliveira, M. M., Gurgel, M. S., Amorim, B. J.,
Ramos, C. D., Derchain, S., Furlan-Santos, N., dos

35. PDQ Supportive and Palliative Care Editorial Board.
Lymphedema (PDQ®): Health Professional Version. 2019
Aug 28. In: PDQ Cancer Information Summaries [Internet].
Bethesda (MD): National Cancer Institute (US); 2002-
. Available from:
https://www.ncbi.nlm.nih.gov/books/NBK65803/

36. Pajero Otero, V., García Delgado, E., Martín
Cortijo, C., Romay Barrero, H. M., De Carlos Iriarte, E., &
Avendaño-Coy, J. (2019). Kinesio taping versus compression
garments for treating breast cancer–related lymphedema: A
randomized, cross-over, controlled trial. Clinical
Rehabilitation, 33(12), 1887-
1897. https://doi.org/10.1177/0269215519874107

37. (PDF) Lymphedema and nutrition: A review.

(2019, May 13). Retrieved from
https://www.researchgate.net/publication/33307
0045_Lymphedema_and_nutrition_A_review

38.   Santos, C. C., & Sarian, L. O. (2018). Long term effects of manual lymphatic drainage and active exercises on physical morbidities, lymphoscintigraphy parameters and lymphedema formation in patients operated due to breast cancer: A clinical trial. PLOS ONE, 13(1), e0189176. https://doi.org/10.1371/journal.pone.0189176

39.   Schwartz, N., Chalasani, M., Li, T. M., Feng, Z., Shipman, W. D., & Lu, T. T. (2019). Lymphatic Function in Autoimmune Diseases. Frontiers in immunology, 10, 519. https://doi.org/10.3389/fimmu.2019.00519

40.   Sugisawa, R., Unno, N., Saito, T., Yamamoto, N., Inuzuka, K., Tanaka, H., Sano, M., Katahashi, K.,

41.   Şener, H. Ö., Malkoç, M., Ergin, G., Karadibak, D., & Yavuzşen, T. (2017). Effects of Clinical Pilates Exercises on Patients Developing Lymphedema after Breast Cancer Treatment: A Randomized Clinical Trial. The journal of breast health, 13(1), 16–22. https://doi.org/10.5152/tjbh.2016.3136

42. Tantawy SA, Abdelbasset WK, Nambi G, Kamel DM. Comparative Study Between the Effects of Kinesio Taping and Pressure Garment on Secondary Upper Extremity Lymphedema and Quality of Life Following

43. Turk J Surg. (2017). Lymphedema: From diagnosis to treatment. DOI: 10.5152/turkjsurg.2017.3870

44. Uranaka, H., Marumo, T., & Konno, H. (2016). Effects of compression stockings on elevation of leg lymph pumping pressure and improvement of quality of life in healthy female volunteers: A randomized controlled trial. Lymphatic Research and Biology, 14(2), 95-103. https://doi.org/10.1089/lrb.2015.0045

45. Wang, J., García-Bailo, B., Nielsen, D. E., & El-Sohemy, A. (2014). ABO genotype, 'blood-type' diet and cardiometabolic risk factors. PloS one, 9(1), e84749. https://doi.org/10.1371/journal.pone.0084749

46. Wanchai A, Armer JM. Effects of weight-lifting or resistance exercise on breast cancer-related lymphedema: A systematic review. Int J Nurs Sci. 2018;6(1):92-98. Published 2018 Dec 24. doi:10.1016/j.ijnss.2018.12.006

47. Zuther, J. E. (2011). Lymphedema Management: The Comprehensive Guide for Practitioners. Stuttgart, Germany: Thieme.